One More Day

One More Day

Sefra Kobrin Pitzele

Illustrations by David Spohn

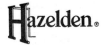

Hazelden®

First published April, 1988.

Copyright © 1988, Hazelden Foundation.
All rights reserved. No portion of this
publication may be reproduced in any
manner without the written permission
of the publisher.

ISBN: 0-89486-519-6

Printed in the United States of America.
Library of Congress Catalog Card Number
88-80363

Editor's Note:

Hazelden Educational Materials offers a
variety of information on chemical dependency and related areas. Our publications
do not necessarily represent Hazelden or
its programs, nor do they officially speak
for any Twelve Step organization.

DEDICATION

One More Day is dedicated, in love and gratitude, to those wonderful people who surround me and who form my personal support system.

To my children — Debbi, Mark, and Amy — for their patience and unflagging faith in me and for their hugs and kisses and for the joy they spread. And to my mom, Esther Kobrin, who believes in me no matter what I do.

To my closest friends, who don't ask how they can help but just help, I send my deepest love and warmest thanks. So, to Dianne Siegel, Nancy Ruvelson, Paula Pergament, Linda Gersick, Vicki Gross, Nancy Gilats, and a cast of dozens more — I love you all.

To my friend Sister Mary Kraemer with special love and blessings for listening, for helping, for being there.

To the editorial staff at Hazelden Educational Materials, special thanks for their patience, kindness, guidance, and skill.

Sefra Kobrin Pitzele

INTRODUCTION

We all pride ourselves in our ability to rise to a challenge, to overcome the odds, and to accept change. One of the changes which can occur is diminished health. Our taken-for-granted good health gives way, often slowly, to aches and pains and other health problems. My first book, *We Are Not Alone: Learning to Live with Chronic Illness*, addresses the many problems we may have when adjusting to long-term health changes.

One out of three people will develop some form of chronic illness, such as arthritis, heart disease, or diabetes. Medical problems often become a permanent part of our days, an increasing change we must adapt to and accept.

We realize that it's not just we who are affected, but all the people — family and friends — who surround us. This book of meditations is for each of us who has experienced changing health or who loves someone who is not always well.

Through this book I pray we each can regain some personal strength to embrace all the goodness and joy life has to offer.

January

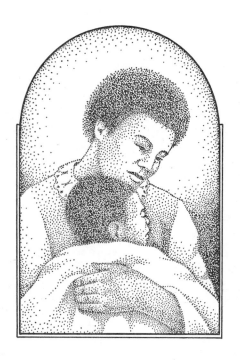

*The beginning is the most important
part of the work.*

> — *Plato*

On occasion we feel a bit sad as we
ready ourselves for bed, knowing that our
bedtime routine marks the end of another
day. We may experience a slight sense
of loss — time lost, opportunities lost, a
piece of life gone forever. Or we may
be filled with regret over words uttered
harshly.

We can put this back into perspective
with the realization that the nicest part
about going to bed at night is knowing
the daylight will come in the morning. We
can't erase today's mistakes, but we can
leave them with the day now past. We can
set our sights on tomorrow. The day we
awaken to will hold a golden opportunity
— to make amends, to make changes, to
use our time well, to start the rest of our
lives anew.

*My life is made of some endings and many
beginnings. I can choose to end an unproductive
pattern by seeing it as a chance to begin.*

January 2

Our share of night to bear,
Our share of morning . . .
　　　　　　— *Emily Dickinson*

We pray for one more day. One more week. Just until the next marker of time or the next major event occurs. "Just let me live until spring," we pray, "until my newest grandchild is born . . . until my next birthday." We pray and may not even recognize these silent, secret pleas as being prayers. It's human nature to ask for a little more time. Most of us feel as though we have not completed our role on earth.

Time, however, is gradually becoming more of a friend than an enemy. We have today, which is all that anyone — healthy or chronically ill — really ever has. No one has an iron-clad promise of weeks, months, or years. Our acceptance of life's unpredictability frees us of our preoccupation with *more* time and allows us to use *this* time — today.

Life is now — today — and I value it by living fully.

Laugh at yourself first, before any-body else can.
— *Elsa Maxwell*

A sense of humor is an essential living tool. Unfortunately, it is most difficult to keep a sense of humor when we're under stress, and that's the time we need it most. In the face of a crisis, we may have found it easier to be dour and nasty, even if we knew, deep in our hearts, that such an attitude was not in our best interests.

Ironically, our medical problems have helped many of us cultivate a humorous attitude toward life. Making the choice between bitterness and acceptance is easier when we take ourselves less seriously. Seeing the funny side of life helps us deal with the most difficult situations life has to offer. Humor cleanses us through spontaneous laughter. It draws others to us and bonds us.

I choose to see humor and lightness in my life. I will allow this attitude to brighten my life and that of those around me.

January 4

Time is a dressmaker specializing in alterations.
— *Faith Baldwin*

Each stage of life brings its own gifts. Every age gives us a chance to examine where we are right now. When we were young, many of us still insisted that we could change the world. We even thought we could change people. The next stage in life may have given us the gift of seeing that we could only change ourselves.

Whatever stage we are in right now is the perfect place to reassess our priorities again. It has become obvious to us by now which things we cannot change, and we are busily accepting that truth.

Time itself alters us and our expectations. The time we have lived has already created change, and the passing of time will create more. The alterations we make today can help us accept this stage in life as being the best place to be.

Now is the time to alter my expectations of myself, to tailor them to my current needs.

*We are never as fortunate or as un-
fortunate as we suppose.*
— *La Rouchefoucauld*

Pain, especially continual pain, is very
draining and is often one of the largest
problems associated with chronic illness.
In the beginning we may have reacted to
our pain with anger or whining and, in
doing so, came to see ourselves as victims
or martyrs. That self-image made us feel
helpless, powerless.

Now, we're better able to understand
pain, not as a curse thrust upon us, but
as our bodies' normal function. Pain, is
a signal and sometimes a warning. But
pain can assist us now in better manage-
ment of our illnesses by helping us regain
some of our personal power and inner
strength. Methods such as relaxation therapy, biofeedback, and self-hypnosis can
all work on different levels to control our
pain. Appropriate exercise can also be an
excellent method of pain control.

I will explore ways to deal with my pain.

January 6

A little learning is a dang'rous thing.
— *Alexander Pope*

Since childhood we've been told that education is the key to success, to happiness, to almost all good things in life. We gradually gain knowledge as we go through school and continue through life, and at each plateau we feel more confident. But a crisis may undermine that confidence. Problems within our families, such as alcohol or other drug abuse or a chronic illness, can sharply point out how little we really know. Our reactions differ — some of us dive into a frenzy of denial and activity, while others are immobilized by fear and uncertainty.

But then we remember: Learning is the key; we don't have to know instinctively what to do. We can turn to others who have greater knowledge. Organizations are there to give us well-qualified assistance. We want and need to learn the truth.

I don't have to have all the answers, just the right questions.

*All human wisdom is summed up in
two words: wait and hope.*
— *Alexandre Dumas*

As children, the only waiting and hoping we did was short-term. We waited for the holidays. We hoped our parents wouldn't find out we got the carpet dirty.

Once a chronic medical problem is diagnosed, we become masters at the art of waiting and hoping. Waiting to see if the new medication helps. Hoping for a remission or cure.

We learn that in order to adjust we must help ourselves. One way we can help ourselves is to get in touch with one of the many self-help groups. These groups can offer us a sense of continuity, of inner strength, of hope for better times again. With deepened faith in ourselves and in our abilities, we discover a sense of inner peace.

Hope renews me and lets me face each day with the best possible attitude.

January 8

*Along with success comes a reputation
for wisdom.*

— *Euripides*

Our definition of success varies as we move through stages of life. While we once may have dreamed of a large lake home and a large salary, we may have settled for a modest home and salary. As we reevaluate our goals, we become aware that we have succeeded in our own way.

Success, for us, might mean we have many friends. Or that our children have become worthwhile citizens. We may feel successful largely because we have learned to accept ourselves — the total package of strengths and weaknesses. We set and reset our own goals throughout a lifetime, and our successes are measured, not by specific deeds or accumulations of cash, but by how well we set our goals and how faithful we are to them.

I'll look again at my values and goals to be sure they leave me room for success.

*Every baby born into the world is a
finer one than the last.*
> — *Charles Dickens*

Place a newborn infant in any adult's
arms, and that adult will turn all attention
to the tiny new life. Most of us feel overwhelmed with the miracle of birth and the
beauty contained within that tiny body. To
hold an infant is to feel perpetuity and an
incredible sense of joy. In the infant, we
see a projection of life and the full scope
of life's possibilities.

Long ago, others marveled at the
fragility and wonder of life as we were
placed as babes in their arms. Now we
recognize we all had the same beginnings,
we all had time before us. We still have
time, and it is still full of possibilities.

*I marvel at the gift of life and all that lies before
me.*

January 10

In loving myself I gain the power of identity that is necessary before love for others is possible.
— David G. Jones

Throughout our lives, we may have loved and cared for other people more than we did for ourselves. Some of us were raised to feel that self-love meant selfish. And some of us had trouble finding anything in ourselves that we could love.

Learning to love ourselves is not easy, especially if our lives are not going the way we had hoped. And those of us who had expected greater personal growth are often unable to take pride in what progress we've made. If we hoped for perfection, we were bound to be disappointed.

Now, we're more likely to see self-love as meaning self-acceptance. We simply offer ourselves what we've so freely offered others — love, care, and a second chance.

I am a worthy person, deserving of love and forgiveness.

Always do one thing less than you think you can do.
— *Bernard Baruch*

Without even realizing it, we all have developed different levels of expertise. Too often, however, our knowledge of ourselves and of our physical capabilities is what we know the least of. The true measure of knowing ourselves, regardless of how capable we seem to be, is to stop the activity before we get too exhausted, before we have too much pain — before we cause an accident.

Understanding one's own body has become a primary concern for many of us because now we realize that how we ''used to'' function doesn't matter anymore. What does matter is how our bodies function right now, and we learn to structure our goals and expectations around those limitations.

I am learning, finally, how to recognize and heed my own body's warning signals.

January 12

> *It's a fine thing to rise above pride,*
> *but you must have pride in order to*
> *do so.*
>
> — *George Bernanos*

We are entitled to feel proud of our accomplishments. Pride is an essential ingredient in the recipe of life, and it comes from an inner sense of well-being, from knowing we have done the best we could under difficult conditions.

When our day's plans are upset by the unexpected, we may struggle with maintaining our pride. We may have been completely independent but now have to rely on others. Or we may have had little pain before and are now overwhelmed by it. Increasingly, we see that we need to find a solution to these new problems or to adjust to those which have none. Solutions and adjustments may be difficult, but we are incorporating them into our lives. We are entitled to feel proud.

Pride is mine as I adjust to my new problems.

We cannot live, sorrow or die for somebody else. . . .
— *Edward Dahlberg*

Our need to protect a sick child becomes frustration as we can do so little to protect the child from pain. When we become ill, our families and friends sometimes make awkward efforts to help protect us. They may try to make us laugh by telling jokes or recounting funny moments we've shared with them. Or these people might become overly helpful, trying to save us some steps or inconvenience.

We understand their need to help us; all of us want to comfort and protect our loved ones as we would a child. However, we are not children, and the maturity we've gained has reversed the roles we play with our family and friends. We can comfort and protect them by laughing with them and by letting them help us, and this becomes a two-way expression of love.

Today, I will allow others to express their love for me.

January 14

Ill health of body or of mind, is defeat.
Health alone is victory. Let all men,
if they can manage it, contrive to be
healthy.

— *Thomas Carlyle*

This message, on the surface, could be upsetting to people who are chronically ill. Can we be sick and healthy at the same time? We learn that we can. Even if we have an ongoing health need, we can still create a new frame of reference which allows us to be as healthy as we can. Rather than letting our problems run us into the ground, we can make the opposite choice.

We can choose balance in our lives, by deciding to put the problem in its place as only one facet of our lives. At the moment we decide, at the moment we make a conscious decision to be a fighter, we will be striving toward wellness once again.

By constructively choosing to keep a strong attitude emotionally and physically, I will be on the road to balanced health.

*The person who tries to live alone will
not succeed as a human being.*
— Pearl S. Buck

We all enjoy going out to dinner or to
a movie. Some of us who are not well,
however, choose to become stay-at-homes.
Our reasons are many, and one big reason
is we don't want to be stared at or singled
out as different. But, in hiding from the
stares, we also hide from ourselves.

We don't want to put ourselves on the
line, but we must if we are to become
''public'' once again. It may mean using
a cane or a brace; it may mean utilizing
some of the fine adaptive living aids in-
vented to help us. It's a hard decision,
but not as hard as being alone and staying
at home.

*It takes tremendous inner strength to venture
from the protective cocoon of my home. I have
the same inner strength as always, and I can use
it to survive tough times.*

January 16

The future is an opaque mirror. Any-one who looks into it sees nothing but the dim outlines of an old and worried face.

— *Jim Bishop*

When we are young, our mirrors reflect our outer appearance. Later, mirrors seem to reflect also the inward self. Worry and joy can etch themselves into our facial expressions; anger or love can gaze out from our eyes. If we have refused to forgive, our bitterness stares back at us. If we have chosen to isolate ourselves, our loneliness is there. But if our choices have been openness, humor, and understanding — all of these clearly shine out for all to see.

Each day, without realizing it, we are making choices for behaviors and thoughts that will help create either a serene and joyful face or an old and worried one. The choice is ours.

Today, I choose healthy looks, actions, and feelings.

Probably no one alive hasn't at one time or another brooded over the possibility of going back to an earlier, ideal age in his existence and living a different kind of life.

— Hal Boyle

If we could go back to a more perfect idyllic life, what section of life would we choose? As we daydream about the wonderful ''yesterdays'' in our life, little do we realize that even though our health and life circumstances may have changed somewhat, we could, right at this very moment, be creating the memories upon which we will look back fondly.

We make our own good times and our own good memories. We can't ever go backward — but we do still have the ability and capacity to move forward.

I am aware that it's up to me to create all my future memories. I can take from life only as much as I am willing to put into it.

January 18

Life's a pretty precious and wonderful thing. You can't sit down and let it lap around you . . . you have to plunge into it, you have to dive through it.

— *Kyle Crichton*

Life isn't always carefree. Especially when we are suffering pain and discomfort, we may tend to back away from the mainstream. We're just not sure how to behave in the face of new problems. We become confused about what is expected of us and what we expect from others. Uncertain of what to do, we may be content for a while to let life lap around us.

We find, however hard the lesson, that in order to be a participant, to get into the swing of things, we must dive back into life. No one is going to take care of all our needs. We are responsible for our actions.

I have been confused how to continue living my life. Now I understand that I must plunge in again and get going.

Wisdom is knowing when you can't be wise.

— *Paul Engle*

Whenever we previously thought of wisdom we may either have imagined a venerated sage or a beloved grandparent. Or we may have thought of formal schooling and college degrees.

We remember wisdom learned from our parents. We remember conveying similar ideas to our children. How many of us really remember the first time we had to answer, ''I don't know''? And what about the moment when it finally occurred to us that there are certain skills that we will never be able to develop?

Understanding comes when we expand ourselves to our fullest capacities and accept ourselves just as we are. Then and only then are we wise.

The more comfortable I become with my limitations, the more I can grow.

January 20

Life is full of internal dramas . . .
played to an audience of one.
        — Anthony Powell

Our lives are filled with dramas. Some of them we were able to talk about to similarly involved people, and some, we found, had to remain private.

Health changes can create hundreds of new dramas. In the beginning far too many of us made the mistake of telling our experiences to anyone who asked. We talked too often, too long, and too much.

We are learning that gentle lesson of who, when, and how much to tell — selectivity. We discover that no one really wants to be always involved in our dramas, in each tiny success or failure. We can keep our own counsel and give ourselves private praise.

I can choose when — and when not — to share some of the dramas in my life.

*Historic continuity with the past is
not a duty, it is a necessity.*
— *Oliver Wendell Holmes*

Our personal histories mark the pathways of life. Our having lived and loved and worked makes a difference in thousands of ways. This impact on life is a history and heritage for our loved ones and for ourselves. What memories have we created for those we love? Perhaps quilts that will be treasured as family heirlooms. A family farm or profession? But what else?

Even more important than heirlooms and family jobs are loving memories and personal histories. Recorded histories, especially anecdotal, can be written or tape recorded. Pictures can be taken, and older photos can be labeled for the generations to come. What will we leave when we die? Communication, tradition, and the ability to love unconditionally.

This small but important moment is a good time to record my journey thus far and to affirm my sense of continuity.

*To live happily is an inward power of
the soul.*

— *Marcus Aurelius*

While we were still very healthy, we
may not have realized how much we depended on others for our physical and
emotional well-being. Perhaps we rarely
turned toward our own strength or to a
Power greater than ourselves. Because we
had depended so little on ourselves, we
may have, at first, felt defeated.

Ironically, we've become strengthened
by illness. Soul searching and taking personal inventory are tools we use to discover the mental and spiritual reserves
that were always available to us but little
used.

The love and support of others are still
important to us, but now we have a greater
sense of balance which strengthens us and
our relationships.

*My inner spiritual messages transcend my need
to depend on others. This strengthens me, my
faith, and all the people touched by my life.*

*Those wrinkles are the map of my life.
. . . They're battle scars.*
— *Etta Furlow*

One woman calls her wrinkles a patina that glows only with age. When first we notice tiny wrinkles — crow's feet or smile lines — we may lament our loss of youth.

Naturally, our faces change as we age. Our life experiences, both joy and pain, etch themselves on our faces as surely as they mold our minds and spirits. Our bodies may begin to change as well. Previously nimble fingers may stiffen; backaches and a slowed pace may become the norm.

Skin is but a wrapping for the inner soul, and the soul's enjoyment of life is not diminished by its wrapping. Our spirits never grow old. Our belief in the beauty and joy of life is renewed with each season. And we remain strong.

My body will change as the years go by, but I will stay aware of my spirit and faith. This keeps me emotionally vibrant.

> *The type of hugging I recommend is the bear hug. Use both arms, face your partner and perform a full embrace.*
>
> — *David Bresler*

We all need physical contact. And this contact does more than put us in touch with other people; it reminds us of our human need to love as well as to be loved.

Some of us may have a sense of aloneness, regardless of how many or few people surround us. If we live alone, it can be most difficult to get our daily ration of hugging and touching. Perhaps we need to consider buying a pet. A bird, a cat, a dog will offer affection all the time. All they require is a good, loving home. Or perhaps we need to think about the contact we have with others. Our expressions of love bring us the unexpected bonus of physical well-being.

I need to love and be loved. I will share my caring nature more freely with other living creatures.

Self-understanding rather than self-condemnation is the way to inner peace and mature conscience.
— *Joshua Loth Liebman*

We can be committees of one, single-handedly striving to show others, by example, that having a chronic medical problem need not keep us out of the mainstream of life. Our health difficulties may heighten our awareness of the value of life, of other people, and of ourselves.

We can hold our heads up high and go out in public. In this way, we refuse to let our diminished health subdue us. By being comfortable with ourselves, smiling at passers-by, and not complaining, we can create an aura of strength and self-assurance. Doing this can challenge and inspire others, and — more importantly — it can do the same for us.

It's difficult sometimes to leave the security of my home. The more I understand my fears, the easier it is to go out among other people.

January 26

*In human relationships, closeness and
warmth only occur when we ask about
one another . . . when we seek to
know how we can help one another.
Until we ask, we will never know.*
— Bernard S. Raskas

Who are our close friends? We should
cherish friendships and protect them as
vigorously as we would a newborn infant.

When a friend comes to us needing
our help, we are forced into making a
decision. One choice — abandonment —
means we lose a friend. The other option
means that the question, ''What can I do
to help you?'' is no longer rhetorical;
it is a commitment to helpfulness. We
may even have to put ourselves at risk,
especially emotionally, but we can be a
friend who stays around when a crisis
occurs.

*I honor my close friendships. I am not someone
who takes and doesn't give personally. I can help
others.*

The ancient sage, who concocted the maxim, "Know Thyself," might have added, "Don't tell anyone!"
— *H. F. Heinrichs*

All too often people hide from their own feelings and from the reality of chronic illness. We may reason that if we ignore it long enough it will go away. Of course, this does not happen, and slowly we gain the knowledge of what our illness is and how we can best live with the changes it creates.

Perhaps we cannot change the course of a chronic illness or medical condition, but we can, and certainly should, change how we react. Bitterness only encourages the company of those who are also bitter. Acceptance, openness, and serenity will attract others who share our willingness to change and grow.

Today, I will be open and honest with myself as I move back into the path of life with an illness at my side.

January 28

Love received and love given comprise
the best form of therapy.
— Gordon W. Allport

Many of us with health problems are — by choice or by necessity — alone, and we may sometimes feel uneasy in a world geared for couples and families. Everywhere there seems to be yet another couple — on a park bench, strolling on the sidewalk, and on television. This is especially painful if we had, at one time in our lives, a happy, long-term relationship.

Now we are finding a more complete and less restrictive sense of companionship and still maintaining our independence. Romantic love is not the only basis for trust and friendship. A friend we can trust may also become a confidante, a strong emotional supporter, and an all-around booster. We may be alone, but we realize that we need not be lonely.

I am lucky to have one close friend. I am blessed when I have several. I am no longer alone.

There is one thing a man cannot change — his parents.
— *David Ben-Gurion*

Sometimes we carry anger for too long and may blame others for our problems. It's time to let go if we have been harboring anger toward our parents or other adults. In our memory, in our perception, they may have harmed us. Regardless of what happened, whether it was imagined or real, we need to let it go.

Unknowingly, we may have developed an attachment to this anger toward our parents, and it may take a professional therapist or a support group to help us break the dependency. We can take responsibility for ourselves and our own behaviors. By no longer blaming our inappropriate actions on anyone else, we can free ourselves of one unhealthy aspect of our lives.

I am attempting to own my life and not see it as an extension of others. Today, I can take responsibility for myself and my actions.

January 30

> *If you make friends with yourself you*
> *will never be alone.*
> — *Maxwell Maltz*

Sometimes, we frantically adopt other people's problems to avoid confronting our own. Hiding from ourselves and our problems solves nothing. Yet some of us are so frightened by the challenge life has thrown before us that we are reluctant to confront it head-on.

Most important is being able to face ourselves, especially when we are alone. We can't always hide in the hustle and bustle of a crowd. But we can find a comfort level within ourselves, regardless of what we face. Then, when our spirituality is deepened and we understand our own struggles — and only then — can we assist, support, and share with others.

My awareness of myself has been enhanced by my new life circumstances. The deeper I dig, the more soul I find. The more soul I find, the more I can share myself.

*I recommend you to take care of the
minutes, for the hours will take care
of themselves.*

— *Lord Chesterfield*

When a lifelong job is over, when
a health problem occurs or mobility
becomes impaired, when family moves
away, the days may become long and
lonely. Then, more than ever, it's important that we take care of our own needs.
Some needs may be immediate, for we
have far more time than we know how
to fill. We may look toward the future,
afraid of all the time that must be filled.

This is a perfect time to reach out into
the community, to begin volunteer work.
There are always people who need us, and
by offering our help we will be helping
ourselves as well. Each day is new and
has new possibilities.

*I refuse to worry about the future or the past.
Instead, I'll try to make a difference today.*

February

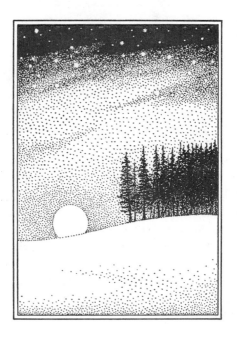

*Snow endures but for a season, and
joy comes with the morning.*
— *Marcus Aurelius*

We are a nation which sometimes sells out for short-term goals and short-term gratification. We may overuse credit cards. At times we live on impulse and buy on impulse. Gone is the long-term planning our parents tried to teach us as children. Gone is learning to wait.

Now we have no choice. Life's circumstances, especially illness, force us to wait whether or not we want to. True, we live with pain and annoyance, but once again, quite accidentally, we begin to know the joy that comes from waiting and from savoring any small victory.

Patience is a virtue I am once again cultivating. Life's circumstances have taught me the importance of finding the joy in each day.

February 2

Every calamity is a spur and valuable hint.

— *Ralph Waldo Emerson*

Events which felt like calamities when we were young have little importance as we get older. Experiences we had labeled ''disastrous'' — not having a date for the prom or failing a math test — now are unimportant or possibly even amusing.

Understanding that many events have only brief importance can help us view current problems more realistically. Not having enough money at the end of the month, family disagreements, and even a flare-up or worsening of a chronic illness are all very important, and they require our attention or adjustment. But we deal with these problems better because we've learned that few, if any, problems are really ''disastrous.'' They're inconvenient or even painful, but our lives can accomodate them. We go on.

I won't see calamities in today's problems and inconveniences.

*Every new adjustment is a crisis in
self-esteem. . . .*

— *Eric Hoffer*

Wouldn't it be nice if our self-esteem
could be as firmly rooted as our personalities seem to have been by the time we
started school? Unfortunately that's not
often the case. Self-esteem is very delicate and remains subject to the whims of
all external circumstances including how
people act toward us and how we react,
in turn, to them.

An illness that changes how we look or
how we think of ourselves can be continually demanding. Fighting the battle to
maintain a good self-image requires adjustments of our time and goals. Making
these adjustments turns our disappointments into chances for success.

*I must continue to work on being a whole person
and try to develop all my facets — spiritual,
emotional, and physical.*

February 4

A simple grateful thought raised to heaven is the most perfect prayer.
— *Gotthold Ephraim Lessing*

Can we picture ourselves as small children, bouncing back out of bed to add just one more, ''and also bless my teddy bear, and my . . .''? Most of us prayed because that's what we were taught to do. We didn't understand many of the reasons, but it felt good and made us feel safe too.

We form new habits as grown-ups. Perhaps prayer isn't part of our day anymore. We may start to pray only when we need to ask for something. It is within our reach to develop the habit of prayer once again. There may be comfort in the habit of giving thanks every day . . . for what good health we do enjoy . . . for the beauty of nature . . . for our family and friends.

I will use prayer as one of the ways I can express myself and live a fulfilling life.

We have seen better days.
— Shakespeare

It is quite difficult to define some of the components that help create what we interpret as a good day. A general sense of well-being prevails, and we have a tendency to look at the world through rose-colored glasses. Everything seems to go just right.

It is not the least bit hard, however, to define a bad day. Nothing happens according to plan. We feel out of sorts, not particularly well. With the advent of health changes, we can inadvertently allow many days to become bad ones.

The only way we can stop having negative experiences is to change our expectations of what constitutes a good day. We don't have to lower our expectations, just make them more realistic for the situation at hand. We will then find that most of our days can be good ones.

My life is and will always be a mixture of good and bad days. I can influence my interactions and thereby influence the color of my days.

February 6

Grow old along with me!
The best is yet to be.
— *Robert Browning*

We all have been to beautiful weddings. A young couple's love is so obvious. They have so much to look forward to, so much living is still ahead.

We understand more and more that now is the best time of our lives. Whether we are having a cup of coffee with a friend or fishing on a quiet lake, these are the best times.

As we age and reach the later decades of our lives, we become aware, even more sharply, that surely these are the best times of our lives. We feel comfortable with ourselves and what we have, and with what we are still accomplishing. We don't set unreasonable goals anymore. And we are lucky, too, for we can blend all our previous years of experience into our daily lives.

I am comforted by knowing that every stage of my life presents me with new opportunities.

Of all sad words of tongue or pen,
The saddest are these: It might have
been.

— *John Greenleaf Whittier*

A story is told of a man leaning over his wife's casket. ''I waited too long,'' he lamented to no one in particular. ''Why didn't I tell her how much I loved her, how much I cherished our life together? I waited too long.''

Like everyone else, we are guilty of procrastination. We tend to put off difficult decisions, such as ending a bad relationship or quitting a job or making amends with an old friend. Our procrastinations seem to protect us.

Now we understand that time is important too. The more we put something off, the less time we have for other more positive areas of life. Life gets easier when we don't procrastinate.

I can resolve many problems with direct actions.
I need not procrastinate anymore.

February 8

Tragedy is an initiation not of human beings but of action, life, happiness and unhappiness.

— Aristotle

Our response to tragedy can be rage, sorrow, or even horror. Those responses, as real as they are, are not as accurate as our optimism, for it is optimism — the belief that life will go smoothly — that gives the label "tragedy" to an event. We are surprised, we are shocked when our optimism is leveled by the unexpected.

A tragedy is an event, a time, a moment, and nothing more. People's lives are constantly see-sawing between emotions and events. No one is always happy, placid, or tragic. In experiencing life to the fullest, we expose ourselves to all its facets. And that simple act makes us all uniquely human.

I accept my life and the ups and downs of my human experience.

A chronic illness invades life.
— *Kathleen Lewis*

Chronic illness means permanently changing our mindset to realize we can move only forward from this point in our life. Chronic illness means pushing back the "front tears" in our mind so we can expand the frontiers of our days. Being ill means sometimes laughing with tears trapped in our hearts, so we won't have to be singled out as different from others. Chronic illness is becoming used to how we look today, right now, and not wasting more time longing for lost yesterdays.

If we haven't realized it yet, we will need more emotional support than perhaps at any other time in our experience. Regardless of how strong and independent we may be, we need comfort and support from those who love us.

Longing for the "old days" and "old ways" won't bring them back. I am learning to accept changes. They are not imposing upon my life — they are my life.

February 10

The best thinking has been done in solitude. The worst has been done in turmoil.

— *Thomas Edison*

When the rush of a busy world becomes overwhelming, we can restore ourselves to peace and tranquility. When we feel battered by the stress of the day, it's time to take a few moments for relaxation. We need to steady ourselves; in fact, we owe it to ourselves.

Solitude, meditation, serenity — these can be ours if we settle in for a few moments of private time. Alone. Taking this time is not self-indulgent; it's self-care and simple to do. We can tune the radio to some beautiful, soft music and sit back with a cup of herbal tea. Taking slow breaths, we can allow our bodies to relax with the warmth of the tea, the beauty of the music, and the solitude of the moment.

I relish the gift of privacy and relaxation each day.

*You are responsible for your own life
and have a job to perform in your
health care.*

— *Neil A. Fiore*

It's a real shock to find out that we have
an ongoing medical problem. Lots of us
may get quite angry and blame the doctor
for the diagnosis. Or we may want to turn
it all over to the professionals. But soon
we begin to see that we are the primary
ones responsible for ourselves. Eventually, we begin to give full cooperation to
our doctors and therapists. We become
equal members of our health-care team.

Adjustments are difficult in the best of
circumstances, but with the help of those
who love us, with the assistance of our
doctors, and with our participation, we
adjust to chronic illness. Then we can see
our problems in their proper perspective
and begin again to enjoy our lives.

*In accepting changes in my life, I find balance
once again.*

February 12

I am where I am because I believe in life's possibilities.
— Oprah Winfrey

During the years of our youth we were continually reminded, ''You can do it. Just set a goal and then reach a little beyond it.'' Many of us were better at this as youngsters than we are as adults. We each have fought our own battles — to become educated or perhaps to achieve a promotion or new job. We tend to get a little short-sighted when a new variable enters the picture — a changing health pattern.

Too many of us back away, fearful that we'll have all we can do to just orchestrate our own health care. It's imperative that we continue to believe in ourselves as human beings with great potential — it matters less that we reach each goal. It matters most that we try.

I am setting new goals that offer challenge and the chance for success.

Joy waits for no man.

— *Tanhuma*

Joyfulness is one of God's greatest gifts. Joy transcends all time and place. Joy causes unmeasurable and often indescribable feelings which we might only have for a fleeting moment. Joy is like opening a special present. It is a state of mind, a frame of reference for future memories.

While we may quite easily recognize the joy of watching an exquisite sunset, we forget too often that it is natural that its beauty changes, dims, and then disappears within moments. And this is true of many of our joy-filled experiences — they change, they dim, and often they disappear. Joy does not always stay with us, so we need to make the most of it when it is upon us — in a sunset, a child's hug, or a friend's offered hand.

To live life to the fullest, I am open to those special moments of joy, even if they don't last forever.

February 14

We don't love qualities, we love persons. . . .

— Jacques Maritain

No matter what happens to us in our lifetime, regardless of whether we are rich or poor, strong or weak, ill or well, we always have room for love. Unqualified love and caring cost nothing. Despite our financial position, allowing ourselves to love, allowing ourselves to be loved strengthens and lends greater value to our lives.

In loving others and in being loved, we are reminded that people, not events or even characteristics, are the important elements of our lives. We don't look for perfection in our loved ones, and we're freed of the notion that we must earn another's love. Love balances our lives; it helps us keep sight of our values and priorities.

I will remember today that I love people for themselves, not for their potential. The love I receive is given just as freely.

*Reality is a staircase going neither up
nor down, we don't move, today is
today, always is today.*
— *Octavio Paz*

Reality is a harsh word and can invade
our everyday lives. When we are struggling to cope with the physical changes
which occur with long-term medical problems, reality becomes our constant companion. No longer can we deny anxiety
or discomfort.

Our self-imposed rules might be the
framework of our lives, but we can build
a new structure which accepts illness as
part of the reality of our lives. This new
structure can have much more depth and
greater dimension than the original, for
we are older and wiser. Part of the framework which gives our days meaning is our
love for friends and family, and recognition of our spiritual capacity. These, too,
become our new reality.

*I no longer expect perfect health, but I can
minimize my complaining and maximize my
efforts to live a meaningful life.*

February 16

Every soul is a melody which needs renewing.

— *Stephne Mellarme*

It may be difficult to admit how discordant our lives become at times — and even more difficult to restore a sense of peace. We may plunge into self-improvement programs with the idea that we, and we alone, can fix ourselves and ease our emotional pain. In doing this, we ignore the spiritual resources outside ourselves.

We better understand and accept our human flaws now and find it easier to ask God for help. Occasionally we may feel inadequate or angry or frightened. We question and doubt ourselves; we get lost in the maze of our own emotions. But we know these feelings are only temporary and that the calming spiritual tempo of our lives is briefly being drowned out by the emotions of the moment. It is comforting to know the melody is always there.

Today, I trust God to keep me in tune with the peace within.

Grace is the absence of everything that indicates pain or difficulty, hesitation or incongruity.
— *William Hazlitt*

It seems that, when we think our lives are back on course, another obstacle appears and we stumble. In the case of physical illness, symptoms or pains may worsen or new problems may crop up. Other circumstances can make our stress level rise as well, until it feels as though we just can't carry the burden anymore.

Adjustments can be very difficult. With new symptoms we may feel that illness is chipping away, one tiny piece at a time, at our independence. It's difficult to be gracious with so many complications going on. Yet this is the time to be gracious — to ourselves and to those around us.

If I have ever needed to reach into my innermost being to find peace and contentment, it is now. I dislike what has happened to my body, but I can continue to be a gracious person.

February 18

Self-pity is our worst enemy and if we yield to it, we can never do anything wise in this world.

— *Helen Keller*

Pity, either from ourselves or others, harms us. Yet, sometimes, we allow it to happen.

What we really need from others is empathy — for them to feel as if they were in our shoes. Pity can be a deep pit to fall into, and the climb back out is difficult. We can't begin to make the ascent until we are fully aware of why we have allowed pity and self-pity to prevail. Maybe feeling sorry for ourselves has been easier than encountering the frustration that may come when we make an effort.

The actions I take today will be based on growth for myself and will help me avoid self-pity.

Arriving at one goal is the starting point to another.

— *John Dewey*

Accepting change in our lives is the basis of growth. Too often, we've seen change as threatening — familiar landmarks are razed, friends move away or die, we become ill.

Eventually, we come to see change in a different light. For good or bad, or whether we approve or don't approve, change will happen. The only thing we can control is our reaction to it. Change that is progress or growth, such as old landmarks disappearing and new ones being built or friends becoming involved in self-help groups, can be welcomed. Other changes which can't be greeted with enthusiasm — losing friends or becoming ill — can at least be seen as random, not personal, consequences of human life. With this frame of mind, we are able to accept the challenges demanded of us.

Changes in my life can encourage growth.

February 20

This is a delicious evening, when the whole body is one sense and imbibes delight through every pore.
— Henry David Thoreau

We carry the memory of a soft spring rain within us even in a dry season. We remember the pungent fragrance of new-mown grass, the chirping of crickets, the singing of birds.

Such memories are important to us, but we're increasingly determined to also create new ones. It takes some planning on our part to get out, but we know the experience is worth the effort. Our mobility may be limited, or we might not be living in a place where we can commune with nature as easily as we did when we were younger. But we're creative and find the joy of outdoors on the stoop of our building or on a park bench. Zoos, nature preserves, and public parks give us areas for today's enjoyment and tomorrow's memories.

My illness imposes real limitations upon me; I will not impose artificial ones upon myself.

I will not keep myself from taking positive action.

— *K. O'Brien*

The inability to get going can sometimes plague us. Muscles that don't work properly or joints that won't bend can keep us from beginning the day as we once did, even if we have excellent intentions.

Excellent intentions only, however, get us nowhere unless we act upon them. What we need is that extra measure of strength, drawn from some inner resource that we hold in store only for days such as these. Often those sources spring from our intense belief that we will make it through these difficult times. Gradually we recognize that our actions and reactions are becoming more positive.

I try to reach a little bit further for the strength I need to fulfill my good intentions.

*The soul would have no rainbow
Had the eyes no tears.*
— *John Vance Cheney*

That familiar tightening in the throat, the welling of tears behind the eyes, and deep emotional pain are all signs of an intense need to cry. Why do we try so hard to be ''brave little soldiers'' and not cry when our bodies are screaming for release?

If we hide behind false smiles and continue to keep the well of emotion untapped, eventually that well will go dry. Deprived of this natural outlet, our minds and bodies exhaust themselves as they battle tension and stress. We lose our ability to express ourselves emotionally. There may be no more opportunity for tears. Tears cleanse and allow other emotions to move in and take over until we need to cry again.

Crying releases me and gives me the freedom to experience my full range of feelings.

Who can separate his faith from his actions, or his belief from his occupations?

— *Kahlil Gibran*

We may, at times, represent ourselves in an untrue fashion. This may happen when we are trying to impress someone who doesn't know us well. We may unconsciously try to imitate another person. Yet in doing so we are not being faithful to the gift of our own uniqueness.

Our need to ''prove ourselves'' diminishes only when self-esteem and self-awareness blossom. As we become more secure, we begin to honestly express ourselves and our faith. We no longer need heroes to worship; we can instead honor the gift of life.

I find comfort in the honest expression of my beliefs and feelings.

February 24

*The future is like heaven — everyone
exalts it but no one wants to go there
now.*
— *James Baldwin*

There are people called futurists who
specialize in studying trends and attitudes
and who then form theories as to what
the future will hold. Having a reasoned
opinion about future needs is important
for business, education, and industry. It's
probably not so important for us. We
work harder to understand today and to
discover what this day can hold for us.

We aren't scientists or researchers; we
are more like explorers who face un-
charted territory. Each morning we're unaware of all the events and surprises that
lie ahead, but we are the only ones who
can choose the direction this day will take.
We don't want to and we don't need to
worry about the future because right now
we have this gift of time to use for ourselves and for those who are close to us.

I will glory in this day and fill it with living.

He who attempts to resist the wave is swept away, but he who bends before it abides.

— *Leviticus*

Just as water transforms the definition of the shoreline, so can our changing health patterns alter the boundaries of our days. What looked and felt normal before may be entirely alien now.

In various stages of life, we've repeatedly demonstrated our ability to adapt to new situations. Marriage, children, new jobs all call for personal change. Add to these everyday occurrences a chronic medical condition (physical or emotional) and we may feel we are drowning. Perhaps at these times, we can disengage ourselves from the moment, reassess the past, and recall how well we've handled the changes life has demanded. We have been adaptable, and we can continue to be.

Creating a new pattern of living is definitely within my reach.

February 26

I shall not pass this way again;
Then let me now relieve some pain,
Remove some barrier from the road,
Or brighten someone's heavy load.
                                    — *Eva Rose York*

Sometimes we help others through — neighborhood clean-up committees, recycling stations, and paint-a-thons. Maybe we've volunteered through school or church or community organizations.

Illness has helped us better understand the relationship between those who help and those who need help. Loving help is not prompted by pity or superiority, but by empathy and shared humanness. Also, we've learned that no one is always the helper or always the one needing help. We are both. We are bonded to others through what we give — and what we receive.

I will show my love by helping and being willing to be helped.

Friendship needs no words — it is solitude delivered from the anguish of loneliness.

— *Dag Hammarskjold*

The meaning of ''pregnant pause'' is clear when we are with close friends. We feel no need to entertain them. There is comfort in the silence.

A friend knows almost intuitively when we have pain and when we do not. A friend lets us ramble on as we try to adjust to a changing lifestyle. We make judgments about how much to share. Even friends can be wearied by an endless litany of complaints. We trust our friends, but we also trust the comfort of silent understanding.

I am thankful for my friends with whom I can share in words and in silence.

> *We all like to forgive, and we all love*
> *best not those who offend us least, not*
> *those who have done the most for us,*
> *but those who make it most easy for*
> *us to forgive them.*
>
> — *Samuel Butler*

None of us likes to harbor angry or bitter feelings toward another person. We know that friends may drift apart because of disagreements in which neither of us will bend or compromise.

More and more, we know what our values are and the importance of how we reflect those values. When a friendship is threatened by anger or misunderstanding, we're able to let our values guide us. We've been less willing to sacrifice our values to save a weak relationship. We've let go of some friends. If we've been stubborn or selfish, we're better able now to preserve the friendship by making amends.

I will nurture my friendships and myself by letting my principles guide my life.

Once you have experienced the seri-
ousness of your loss you will be able to
experience the wonder of being alive.
— *Robert Veninga*

Age and illness force us to come to
terms with the sometimes harsh reality
of being human. When someone close
to us dies, we may be overwhelmed with
sadness. We might grieve over and over
until it seems we can grieve no more. And
then we begin to heal. Granted, it takes
time and a good bit of faith, but we do
recover. Slowly. One day at a time.

Many of us have experienced sorrow
over changes in our health. With time and
faith, however, we're learning that the
anger and sadness also heal. And eventually we recognize that our experience has
made us more sensitive, more caring, and
more receptive to the gift of life.

I will grieve my losses and then move, once
again, into a fulfilling, joyful life.

March

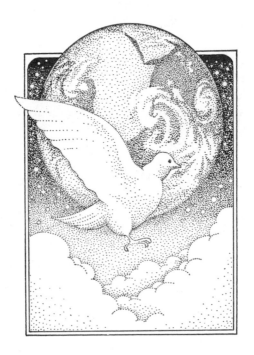

There is no way to peace. Peace is the way.

— *A. J. Muste*

So often we look for easy answers and quick remedies. We want to reach our goals — now. Whatever we're looking for (peace, love, acceptance) we may be making the mistake of seeing these qualities as concrete, hold-in-my-hand goals.

Gradually, we're coming to the understanding that those qualities we seek are not destinations; they are paths and directions we can consciously take. We can't go out and find love, but we can choose to be loving. There is no path to peace or to acceptance or to understanding, but we can base our lives on these qualities, and by doing so we claim them.

What I seek may already be within my soul.

March 2

Bitterness and anger seem to be very closely related and are interchangeable words for the same emotion.
— *Robert Lovering*

Why me? We may rage with anger or disbelief when we finally realize we may never fully regain good health. In the beginning, while we are still getting used to our new situation, this happens to most of us. And then we ask, ''Why me?''

Having a chronic medical condition is not as likely to create bitterness as much as making poor choices about how to respond to it. If we choose loneliness or a lifestyle which allows no room for laughter, we choose bitterness.

By making healthier choices, we affirm our belief in ourselves, in the possibilities life has to offer. We feel more loving toward the people around us and, in doing so, are more loving toward ourselves.

I can learn to balance my negative feelings with contentment and happiness. I can gain strength from my illness.

*People, by and large, will relate to the
image you project. . . . If you project
the image of a sick, dependent person,
that's how you'll be treated.*
— *Chyatte*

Accepting chronic illness is not easy.
Our whole lives are different. We can't
do all the things we used to do. We may
feel changed and be afraid of the changes
our illnesses will bring. But as we learn to
project a strong, positive image, we feel
better about ourselves.

For the benefit of ourselves, we must act
as if we are doing all right. When we act
as if we are strong, our new behavior can
become a new habit, and that habit can actually develop greater emotional strength
within us. We can put illness into perspective as being just one of the changes
that occur during a lifetime.

*Today, I will allow myself the right to change. I
can survive my health change and live a worthwhile life.*

March 4

Whatever limits us, we call fate.
— *Ralph Waldo Emerson*

We like to plan ahead, but we cannot plan for the ravages of chronic illness. No one expects to travel down the winding road of an unbidden, unwanted trip. Unused to the whims of a chronic illness, we may at first try to chart, plan, and control its course. We may dwell too much on our medical conditions.

We cannot change the course of illness, but we can influence its twists and turns by keeping a positive frame of mind. Rather than being obsessed with how our medical conditions are affecting us, we can focus on the many things we can still do. Can we enjoy a sunset? Watch a child smile? Can we listen to music or pursue a handcraft? Our angry, dour thoughts can be replaced so easily with pleasant dreams, fond memories, and hope for the future.

I am feeling comfortable once again as I finally realize that I can still make choices in how I want to live my life.

*Our sweetest songs are those that tell
of saddest thoughts.*
— *Percy Bysshe Shelley*

Our inner messages are much like tuning a radio; we choose what we want to hear. With a turn of the radio dial, the music changes from mellow and happy to sad and lonely and back again.

The inner messages we choose to hear may fill our days with memories that are difficult to bear. But we can tune our minds to more positive thoughts, by noticing the beauty of our surroundings, by focusing on more pluses and on fewer minuses. We can, willingly, switch our minds to thoughts that are better for us and for our health.

Why should we listen to the sad, lonely sounds when we have other choices? We can choose a daily program to suit our goals and needs, one that enhances desires and improves general well-being.

Today, I will turn my personal dial to more positive messages.

March 6

The unfortunate thing about this world is that good habits are so much easier to give up than bad ones.
— Somerset Maugham

Old habits often die hard, especially bad ones. We may need to be tactfully silent when we become irritated with the behavior or habits of our loved ones. It may seem at times as though everyone around us is either nail biting, smoking, cussing, or overeating. When illness enters the scene, or any other stressor for that matter, bad habits tend to resurface. We may be less tolerant of others' faults and even of their good health.

It's hard to put away old habits, especially the old pattern of being critical, but we can learn to let go. Even with extra stress in our lives we can begin to work on developing new habits. We can learn to recognize the growth we've achieved and to feel proud.

I can begin today to develop strong, new habits and to hold on to my old, strong habits.

*Life if you will, is a work of art, and
if we have paid loving attention to its
details, we will be able to take pride
in the finished product.*
— *Harold Kushner*

Without even realizing it, we often do
things that are good for us and make
us happy. We do something that creates
well-being, and we have a successful day.
When we pay attention to actions that
create well-being we can have a successful
week. Taking good care of our homes
makes us feel proud and so does helping
a fellow human being in need. Making
volunteer work a part of how we live,
showing kindness to others and ourselves,
reaching out — all these choices enhance
our well-being.

When we pay attention to those around
us, a transformation occurs within our
spiritual selves. Then we shall have given
ourselves the gift of a meaningful life.

*I will pay loving attention to the details of my
day.*

March 8

We cannot learn without pain.
— *Aristotle*

It is said that pain and experience are life's two greatest teachers. What good would it be if we felt pain each day but never learned from it? And what good would it be if we coasted through life without experiencing joy along with sorrow?

There can be no depth of personality or depth of character if our lives have been perfect. Experience etches our hearts and souls, gives us depth, and deepens the horizon of our days. No individual has lived a life completely without pain, without sorrow. We can move beyond our pain and sorrow to grow in new directions.

I can accept the lessons I am learning of tolerance to living a less-than-perfect life. These lessons help me grow.

Don't waste today regretting yester-
day instead of making a memory for
tomorrow.

— *Laura Palmer*

Our youthful dreams were filled with grand expectations of our impact on the world. Some of those goals were reached; many were not.

Now, it's easier to accept that not all our plans will come to pass. In accepting that, we are able to set new goals that better reflect our dreams and ideals today. For a while it may seem as though we are ''just surviving,'' but we can have more.

At our stage of life we are capable of making mature decisions, of setting more realistic goals. Each day we can reflect upon our accomplishments and upon the joy of family, friends, and job. Finally, we can feel comfortable with ourselves, and we can look forward to our tomorrows.

Yesterday is gone and unchangeable, but today
is real and is mine to use.

March 10

You cannot teach a man anything.
You can only help him find it within
himself.

— Galileo

We can't avoid the crises, large or
small, that are a normal part of living. Au-
tomobile accidents, spending more money
than we can afford, stubbed toes, rain on
vacations — these things happen to everyone. No one is exempt. But we can learn
from our negative experiences. We learn
to be more careful, to hold our tongues,
to be more responsible.

No one can teach us how to live. We
have to learn by ourselves. And eventually
we're better able to handle our own problems, sometimes even with grace and fi-
nesse. We can share what we have learned
with others, we can help pave the way for
them, but invariably they too will have to
do it for themselves.

Life hands me situations. I have the ability to
make them into positive experiences.

*The hopeful man sees success where
others see failure, sunshine where others see shadows and storm.*
— *O. S. Marden*

Once in a while we lose sight of the
world around us and get caught up in how
miserable we are feeling. We may be in
physical or emotional pain and become
self-absorbed. Or we may be unhappy
because things are not going exactly the
way we want.

But we can imagine, just for a moment,
a beautiful watercolor picture of a sunrise
— the promise of a brand-new day. The
hues are gentle pastels. The colors blend
together subtly, gently, with no percep-
tible break from one section to another.
We can relax in the beauty and serenity
of the scene. We can enjoy it with no
other motive than pleasure. Positive imagery can help us enhance the beauty of
the moment.

*I am overwhelmed by nature's beauty and by
the great joy I feel. I can call back these same
feelings by visualizing them in my mind.*

March 12

Never bend your head. . . . Look at
the world straight in the face.
— *Helen Keller*

Pride is elusive when we're hurting emotionally. We may act and feel overwhelmed. It is very difficult to be mindful of all we can accomplish and we may focus on what is out of our reach. Or we may tend to hide from our problems by withdrawing from social gatherings or by isolating ourselves emotionally. Feeling ashamed that we are hurting makes asking for help very hard.

Now, as we hide less often from our feelings, we find it easier to face the world straight on. We may not have made this transition easily or even by ourselves, but we are making it with the help of loving friends. Increasingly, we accept our limitations, make the effort to do what we can, and ask for help when we must. And with this, we raise our heads with pride.

I need not be ashamed when I must ask others
for help.

*The longer I live the more beautiful
life becomes.*
— Frank Lloyd Wright

When we were younger, day and night were two separate entities. Day was when we played, and night was when we slept. The distinction is not that sharp as we get older, expecially if we have any problems which disturb our sleep. Worry and pain have a tendency to make nights much longer — and lonelier.

What looked hopeless the night before can take on a whole new light in the morning. It would be wonderful if we could learn to treat each new day with the same freshness we had as children. We can learn, once again, to experience and to savor each moment. Once we separate night and day, the way we did years ago, the more likely we are to allow ourselves wonderful days again.

My expectations are that I will achieve the best each day has to offer.

March 14

*A cheerful face is nearly as good for
an invalid as healthy weather.*
— *Benjamin Franklin*

Health changes, like other changes in life circumstances, can undermine friendships. When we are dealing with chronic pain or discomfort or when we have become impaired with illness, some friends just aren't sure how to act under the new circumstances.

People who love us want to help us; they want to be with us. The hard part for us is how to let them. Visits won't be easy for us or them at first because our lives and relationships are changed by illness. But soon we realize that we still care for and need these special people and that we want to show our affection, during the trying times as well as during the better times.

I can find comfort and stability by maintaining my friendships.

*A man without a plan for the day is
lost before he starts.*
— *Lewis K. Bendele*

Some mornings we are tempted, especially when we are having more than our usual share of pain, to resist the demands and responsibilities of the day before us. We are enticed by the thought of making a cup of coffee, climbing back into bed with the newspaper, and hiding from the world.

Although tempting, this is usually not a good plan for us, and what we need is a plan that encourages us to live the day fully. We may actually have to contrive a plan to push us into action. Personal care, chores needing to be done, letters or phone calls to friends, a trip to the store for groceries — these emphasize our importance and the importance of the day. Without a plan, we risk wasting twenty-four hours in loneliness and self-pity.

*I and this day are important, and my plan
reflects this.*

March 16

*Time ripens all things.   No man's
born wise.*

> — *Cervantes*

One moment in time, a phrase from an old song that still rings true. In a single moment we could decide the balance of how we will live our lives. Split-second decisions, not all good ones, permeate the fabric of our lives, of everyone's lives — regardless of medical problems.

Sometimes we are very sorry about a decision we made too quickly, a decision which may alter the course of our lives for a short while or even permanently. Perhaps the car we insisted on having is a lemon, or we may not like the new community into which we impulsively moved. We have to learn to live with our decisions, at least until we make a decision to change. Ponder a decision just a moment longer. Each experience can deepen our wisdom.

I will attempt to take my time when making decisions.

*Time is lost when we have not lived
a full human life, time unenriched by
experience, creative endeavor, enjoyment, and suffering.*
— *Dietrich Bonhoeffer*

''I'll never make it through today!''
While we all may have had that thought
from time to time, we did live through that
day to rise the next morning and greet the
new day. Time can go by very slowly when
we are thinking of no one but ourselves.
Sometimes we can feel overwhelmed by
fear of an uncertain future. We may even
feel that we have been deserted by our
friends and family in a time of need.

When overwhelmed with these helpless
feelings, we can turn to our Higher Power
for comfort and understanding. Knowing
we don't have to work through the details
of our lives alone not only comforts us,
it fills our minutes and days with positive
thoughts and actions.

*My Higher Power lends me strength to carry me
through.*

March 18

*An ordinary man can surround him-
self with two thousand books . . . and
thenceforward have at least one place
in the world in which it is possible to
be happy.*

— *Augustine Birrell*

A flashlight. A winter storm. Secretly
reading under the covers. As children,
most of us escaped into books from time
to time. Books were a private experience,
shared with no one. They could also be a
warm family time of sharing.

Books still provide a window to the
world, to adventures and faraway places
that few people ever experience firsthand.
Regardless of physical ability — or disability — we can generally find a way to read
or listen to a book. We can shed, for a
short while, some of the frustrations we
experience. We can forget the ravages of
illness. We can travel. We can dream.

Reading is a true gift which I can give myself.

*Faith in a holy cause is to a consid-
erable extent a substitute for the lost
faith in ourselves.*

— *Eric Hoffer*

Busy! Busy! Busy! We might feel as
though we're living our lives on a treadmill — always on the go, helping, and
giving our time to people and causes.

Service and volunteerism can be wonderful ways to help, but only if they
augment an already full life. We truly
are living on a treadmill if our involve-
ment is an escape from facing our innermost thoughts and fears. We are getting
nowhere if our outside activities are all we
have to wake up for each morning.

We begin to change when we honestly
face our greatest fears. We can search our
personalities to find our vulnerable points
and then strive to correct what defects we
can. It is then that we regain faith in
ourselves and in our abilities.

*Once I regain faith in myself I can open my heart
to help others.*

March 20

*Understanding human needs is half
the job of meeting them.*
— *Adlai Stevenson*

We may have needed constant reminding to do our chores when we were children. We expected to be told what to do.
Today we are adults and are chronically ill,
and we find ourselves giving reminders to
the people around us. Now, however, the
suggestions have to be extremely delicate
and carefully given.

We can gently guide the behavior of
spouse, friends, parents, and children re-
garding our medical problems. Our com-
ments can be honest and direct: "It would
help me if you would let me try to do
things for myself before offering me your
help." Or "Please sweep the floor."
Or "Would you put the towels into the
dryer?" Those around us are not able to
read our minds. We can learn to say "I
need" or "I want." Our needs will be
met if we ask directly.

Learning to ask for help is hard, but I can learn.

It is a happy talent to know how to play.
— *Ralph Waldo Emerson*

As the carefree days of childhood give way to adulthood, we sometimes forfeit too much of the child. We become what we think is mature — serious and busy. Quite unintentionally we might become caught up in the importance of being married, working hard at our jobs, raising children, or paying off the mortgage. Even at home we might be rushing here and there — mowing the lawn, getting a haircut, buying clothes or groceries, and performing all the small household chores which need doing regularly.

Where is the time we need for ourselves, to spend with friends, or just to play? We can find time, right now, if we want to. We can momentarily shrug off the demands of home or career and lend ourselves to carefree play.

It's sometimes easy to be too serious. Today, I will let myself participate in play.

March 22

Courage is the resistance to fear, mastery of fear, not absence of fear.
— *Mark Twain*

So many of us suffer from flagging self-esteem. This may occur for many reasons, all complex. When we finally decide we are going to create change in our lives, we may be uncertain as to how to make the change. How do we start? One of the best starting places is to adopt one premise of the Twelve Step programs and begin to act ''as if'' we have all the confidence in the world, ''as if'' we have great faith in ourselves. We start to spend time thinking about the possibilities, rather than the impossibilities.

We all fear the unknown, but to act ''as if'' helps us deal with the things we can't see. Eventually, contrived as it feels, our new behavior will become a new habit, and we won't need to act ''as if'' — because we truly ''are.''

I am willing to try to act ''as if'' I can create change.

*There the weary cease from troubling,
and there the weary be at rest.*
— *Job 3:17*

We never thought we would have to learn to live with constant weariness. Our notions of illness may have prepared us for pain, inconvenience, maybe even some negative emotions like anger, but we had no way of anticipating the unrelenting drain of illness. There is tremendous comfort just in knowing we are not alone, that ultimately there is a Power greater than ourselves to whom we can turn for comfort and strength.

We can't always escape the physical weariness of illness, but we can regenerate our spirituality, which may have dissipated along with our good health.

I cannot control my illness, but I can have a hopeful attitude.

March 24

Our safety is not in blindness, but in facing our danger.
— Johann Cristoph Schiller

Sometimes our difficulties are compounded when we take more drugs than needed to treat our illnesses. This can be due to our getting prescriptions from more than one doctor or from using over-the-counter drugs in addition to our prescribed medications.

Certainly, we need to use the drugs that will keep us as healthy and functional as possible, but overmedication can be an accidental side-effect of chronic medical problems. Also, psychological or physical dependence can also occur.

Besides necessary medications, the joy of living and the love of ourselves and others can help us deal with our illnesses. By learning to live with our limitations we can gain back some of the personal power that chronic illness has taken from us.

I am strengthened by facing my problems.

Every man takes the limits of his own field of vision for the limits of the world.

— Arthur Schopenhauer

It's not easy to get used to the idea of a ''forever'' kind of illness. When we first learned about it, we may have allowed it to overtake our lives. Perhaps we lost the pleasure of taking a walk, playing a card game with friends, or spending time helping others. We were obsessed with the memory of how life used to be.

We can learn to put illness into its correct position. We have the chronic condition; it doesn't own us. We will know we have reached true acceptance when the medical issue doesn't dominate our days.

Of course a chronic illness affects us, but now we can see it properly as only one facet of our lives. We can choose to once again have full and meaningful days.

I — not my illness — can choose how well and how fully I will live my life.

March 26

This confrontation with death . . .
makes everything look so precious, so
sacred, so beautiful, that I feel more
strongly than ever the impulse to live
it, to embrace it, and to let myself be
overwhelmed by it.
— *Abraham Maslow*

When we are ill, we are forced to face
our own mortality. A close brush with
death is enough to put the fear of dying
into us, but with this fear a sense of spirituality may flow through our lives. Problems, which once seemed overwhelming,
diminish in size. The trees are greener;
the sky is bluer. People are kinder and
more sharing than ever before.

We often don't miss what we've taken
for granted until it's nearly yanked away
from us. All of a sudden, every day is
a gift. Every day is a precious chance to
live.

I am continuing the struggle to make each day
the best one because I rejoice in the gift of life.

*Patience is the best remedy for every
trouble.*

— *Plautus*

We are used to the quick fix. Candy bars
hold back our hunger. Credit cards allow
us to spend freely when we are financially
strapped. We drive through the fast-food
lanes and eat on the way to our next stop.

And when we were told about our illness, our reaction may have been, ''Okay.
Now how can it be fixed?'' We were told
that part of the treatment was time, a remedy requiring patience and one difficult to
accept. We are learning to accept that the
nature of our illness requires us to be patient. We can use this patience to slow
our often frantic behavior and to notice
the value in each passing minute. Our
time becomes more and more precious as
we understand that patience is a very good
remedy.

Today, I can begin to practice patience.

March 28

> *It is not death or pain that is to be dreaded, but the fear of pain or death.*
> — *Epictetus*

The pain we anticipate — whether it be a flu shot, a lengthy dental procedure, or surgery — is usually worse than the actual pain. Perhaps this is because the anticipation of pain includes fear or dread.

As we deal with pain, we may find healthier ways to cope with it. Once, even the sense of a headache coming might have caused us to tense our muscles and prepare for the onslaught. Now, we're more likely to settle down to begin thinking of positive imagery or relaxation therapy. We are giving ourselves the moments we need to be alone, to breathe deeply, to think of a beautiful and calming sight. We're learning to relax and be less fearful.

I need to remind myself of my personal power. I can exercise control over my body and strive to minimize the effects of fear.

*Happiness should not depend on
physical wellness.*

— K. O'Brien

Without even recognizing that we have
done so, we sometimes structure our entire lives on the foundation of good health.
We assume good health for our future.
And we refuse to even acknowledge that
nature's somewhat random selection process can change the way we live. We may
never even give a moment's thought to
changing our habits because of illness. We
feel exempt, confident it will never happen
to us.

And when it does and our lifestyle
changes — sometimes gradually, sometimes abruptly — we feel we've lost the
right to happiness. Then we begin to adjust. Family and friends stick with us, and
an awareness comes forth that they, not
physical activity, are the reasons for true
happiness.

*I accept and will adjust to chronic illness. Poor
health has changed my life, not ended it.*

March 30

*If you don't learn to laugh at trouble,
you won't have anything to laugh at
when you grow old.*

— *Ed Howe*

Laughing with others is important. Learning to laugh at our own problems, however, is even more important. Since we will continue to live with situations that cause us all types of problems, we may as well learn to laugh at ourselves.

Often with chronic illness, coordination changes. Reaction time may be slower. Sensitivity to cold, heat, or pain may be altered. It's only logical that we will find ourselves in potentially embarrassing situations because of our bodies.

Often, a hearty laugh at all the strange situations flung our way is just the thing to help us work through what is painful and difficult. Laughter is a gift we give to ourselves. We can carry it with us wherever we go, and it will always be ours.

I am headed in the right direction when I can laugh.

Why, why, why?

— James Joyce

"It doesn't seem fair," we privately lament. "How could I have this rotten medical condition just when I've hit my stride — the prime time of my life?"

That's a question we all wonder about. Many of us may get down on our knees and pray to our Higher Power for understanding. We might ask, "Why me?" We might implore, "Why now, when I'm nearly on my feet again?"

We might ask these questions, yet often there are no answers. Our ways are not His ways. Sometimes life just isn't fair; there are no easy answers.

I have adjusted to other changes in my life, and I can adjust to this one too. It may take some time, and I may go through the gamut of emotions first, but I am willing.

April

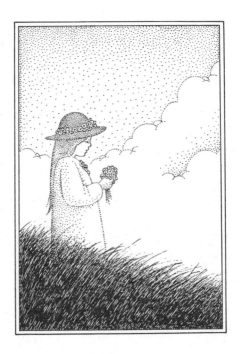

*Spring is a happiness so beautiful, so
unique, so unexpected, that I don't
know what to do with my heart.*
— *Emily Dickinson*

Remember the sheer joy of spring during childhood? How we would race around the backyard, checking out the wonderful sights and smells. Spring in those days meant no more snow pants and boots. It meant being able to dash out with just a light sweater and no admonishments from Mom. And most importantly, the new season heralded a few short months until summer vacation.

We can recapture our youthful openness, for that child is still within us. We can smell the same scents, experience the same joy, but with the depth of understanding we have gained as adults. Regardless of our level of independence, regardless of whether we can plant the garden or just enjoy its flowers, spring can still delight us.

*My heart still delights in spring. I am grateful
to be here to absorb it all.*

April 2

> *The joy of life is to put out one's power in some natural and useful or harmless way. There is no other, and the real misery is not to do this.*
> — *Oliver Wendell Holmes, Jr.*

If our health changes and fatigue are frequent problems, we may become unable to do all we did for ourselves in the past. If we push ourselves too far, something will suffer. We may pay with sore joints or we may pay with depression. But we do pay.

If we liken our daily energy level to money in a bank account, we realize we can make only so many withdrawals before our resources run out. We decide each day how we want to spend — or waste — that precious energy. It takes a while to get our priorities rearranged, but living a good life is important, and eventually we learn how to invest our energy well.

Each day presents itself new and fresh. It's up to me to decide how to spend my energy.

Excessive fear is always powerless.
                                    — Aeschylus

Something may be interfering with our sleep. Eyes wide, we lie in bed night after night. We move through the days like robots, just getting by. Our lack of sleep may stem from worries and problems that we can't face.

Our confrontation with illness may have suddenly made us see how powerless we are over some parts of our lives. Where once we had felt that everything had an acceptable answer, we now have to live with an answer we don't like and we can't change. We may pull that original sense of helplessness into other areas of our lives. Gradually, we understand that life has always been unpredictable; we just refused to see it until we were forced to. We learn to accept the things we can't change and work toward changing the things we can. We deal with our problems. Our anxiety subsides. We're able to rest.

Today, I'll accept unchangeable answers.

April 4

*The mind leaps, and leaps perhaps
with a sort of elation.*
— *Joseph Wood Krutch*

A chronic medical problem can be incorporated into our total picture of life. If we allow problems, medical or otherwise, to overwhelm and exclude everything else, we are defeated before we begin. We don't have to be defeatists.

Every day dawns fresh with opportunities to change, to find happiness, and to live our lives well. By searching deeply within, we can redefine our faith in ourselves and in our Higher Power. A joy, an elation, can be ours when we allow ourselves to express our natural human curiosity through growth, learning, and a willingness to try new things. We can hold our heads up high and be proud.

Regardless of my physical condition, I have dignity and worth.

Be not afraid to pray, to pray is right.
Pray, if thou canst with hope, but
even pray.

— *Hartley Coolidge*

''Now I lay me down to sleep'' may have been one of our first childhood prayers, perhaps even one of our first memories. As we grew, we may have learned to recite other prayers by rote, with little understanding.

Now, we are beginning to understand and feel the need for prayer. Many of us came to a belief in a Power greater than ourselves, one which can nurture and sustain us. We can pray for those we love; we can pray for ourselves. Prayer can enhance and bond us with our Higher Power. It nourishes and satisfies our soul — the inner self.

Prayer is a creative expression of my spiritual needs. It offers me a deep sense of personal satisfaction and continually reminds me of all life's forces.

April 6

*The man who makes no mistakes does
not usually make anything.*
— *Edward John Phelps*

We feel so vulnerable when we have a
chronic illness, almost as though we are
specimens, displayed as oddities. Because
of our vulnerable feelings, we may be
reluctant to undertake new experiences out
of fear that we may expose ourselves to
ridicule. Yet, actually, few people take
the time or trouble to stare.

Living a sequestered life and taking no
chances is not the answer. There are
always options available to us, but they
may be different options from those we
previously considered. We can decide to
take new directions. The image we show
to others is a reflection of the image we
carry within.

*Trying to reach past my mistakes into new suc-
cesses enhances my life.*

Sometimes I have believed as many as
six impossible things before breakfast.
— Lewis Carroll

While sitting at the table with an early morning cup of tea or coffee, we can get lost in reverie. Briefly, for a frozen moment in time, we can believe that we are capable of anything once again.

We still have the joy of our imagination, and even if there are physical restrictions placed upon us by our long-term medical condition, we can still imagine ourselves achieving an impossible dream. It's wonderful to get lost in pure fantasy about how we would like our lives to be. We can imagine ourselves richer in relationships and in friends. Even when our body betrays us, we need never betray the belief in ourselves.

I have the freedom to imagine whatever I want.
My illness doesn't restrict what I can accomplish
in my mind.

April 8

*Believe me, every man has his secret
sorrow, which the world knows not,
and oftentimes we call a man cold
when he is only sad.*
— Henry Wadsworth Longfellow

Let a person seem aloof or display a
need to be apart from others, and we
automatically assume we are getting a cold
shoulder. Yet none of us has any idea
of all the components of another person's
life and feelings. We're usually ignorant
of other people's personal characteristics.
Sadness, shyness, and fear are just a few
traits which can be misinterpreted.

Little disappointments, large failures,
loss of a dream or a loved one — these
are all problems which any one of us can
have, but few can share. We can choose
to overlook the real and imagined wrongs
of others by reminding ourselves of how
little we really know of each other.

*My understanding of other people's problems has
been enhanced by my own illness, and I will not
be so quick to judge.*

The comforter's head never aches.
— Italian Proverb

Sometimes, people who undergo a family crisis, such as the sudden death of a loved one, hold up commendably during the most difficult times, only to collapse later. While none of us can always stay calm, we rarely buckle when our strength is needed by others.

We comfort our loved ones when they're angry, hurt, or disappointed. We comfort friends who have undergone surgery or had other crises of their own. We sit by the bed of people we love as they wait to die. Again and again, we prove we are strong. Our experience in comforting others helps us recognize the strength of our friends and family when they comfort us in our anger or disappointment, in our sadness or illness.

I am proud I can give comfort and strength to those who need it. I am grateful for those who comfort me.

April 10

A friend is a person with whom I may be sincere. Before him, I may think aloud.

— *Ralph Waldo Emerson*

We may wonder what has happened to old friends we have lost touch with over the years. Sometimes we get so caught up in our busy lives we neglect our friendships.

We can rebuild or strengthen a relationship by taking the first step in reaching out to others. Old connections can be reestablished. They were important to us at one time in our lives and can be again. We may find they have been wondering about us as well.

Today, we can take up pen and paper and write to them about ourselves. Now is the time to find out what has happened to our old friends and let them know they're in our thoughts.

I will try today to establish contact with an old friend.

*When you get into a tight place, and
everything goes against you, till it
seems as though you could not hold on
a moment longer, never give up then,
for that is just the place and time that
the tide will turn.*
— *Harriet Beecher Stowe*

Sometimes we push ourselves too fast,
too far, too often. Even though we are
cognizant of that exact moment when we
just cannot, physically or emotionally, go
on any longer, we still persevere.

When we finally do acknowledge that
once again we have gone too far, it may
be time to take a nap or exercise to release our emotions. Or we may choose to
be with friends or family. We begin to
understand that the bad times pass.

If we can just make it through one more
moment, then the tables will turn in our
favor.

*I am able to make it through even the hardest
hard day.*

April 12

A crisis event often explodes the illusions that . . . anchor our lives.
— *Robert Veninga*

Chronic illness can become so commonplace for us that we lull ourselves into thinking we've become the best we can be and believing we can handle everything. When another crisis occurs — family problems, financial setbacks, or loss of friends — we may stubbornly try to fix the situation, only to be rewarded with self-pity or anger or sadness.

In time, we usually realize that we don't have to carry every burden or solve every problem. Sometimes there is no answer other than acceptance of a situation as being unchangeable. What can be changed is our reaction to this fact. We can, as we have before, build our lives around the new situation. We can allow ourselves to grow into a greater maturity.

Every day, every experience is an opportunity to grow.

Tears are summer showers to the soul.
          — Alfred Austin

All our lives, we have been told that time would heal all wounds — and that if time couldn't, then the doctor would.

There are few things which may feel as final as a diagnosis of chronic illness. Chronic means forever — and we can hardly conceive of a problem that will never go away. We may find ourselves crying over and over again, and wonder if the tears will ever end.

For many of us, our tears were how we began to grieve. Grief was how we started to heal ourselves emotionally from the burden of "forever." The tears we shed helped cleanse our thoughts and bodies so we could move on to live the rest of our lives. Today, our grief and weeping will help us continue to grow.

I can let myself shed the purifying tears that well up in my heart. They will help me move on with my life.

April 14

You are the handicap you must face.
You are the one who must choose your
place.

— *James Allen*

Each of us carries a handicap, although
some handicaps are more obvious than
others. They can be physical limitations,
but they can also be emotions, feelings, or
attitudes that impede the full enjoyment
and promise of living. A handicap may
be an image problem or dismay at how
we walk or talk, or it could be chronic
illness. And we certainly can have more
than one handicap.

A full life depends on our ability to cope
with our difficulties and to decide whether
any of them are self-imposed. We haven't
chosen all our limitations — physical or
emotional — but we can choose to strip
our lives of the ones we've created. And
we can choose how we will respond to the
others.

I will define my special place in the world, and
I will try to meet my own best expectations.

Just because everything is different,
doesn't mean anything has changed.
                    — Irene Peter

Change may happen gradually without our being aware of it. A sudden event may force us to recognize how different our lives have become. Yet even when the details or circumstances have changed, we may discover that the real meaning of our lives has remained the same.

We still carry many of the same values as before. We are thankful for the stable relationships that have grown as we have become stronger. We still strive to succeed in the goals we've set. We continue to look for — and to find — meaning in our life experiences. Certainly, we've changed and many things are different, but we continue to carry within ourselves the unique person we each are, the person we've always been.

I have always been a person capable of tremendous growth. I'm thankful that I can make changes that will help me grow.

April 16

*Any real progress in the tangled world
of emotions must be made by the
individual. Each of us must hold
the mirror to our own soul and gaze
intently at what we see there.*
— *Bernard S. Raskas*

"Making do" is an old-fashioned
phrase that signifies our ability to manage with whatever we have. We have all
thought of that phrase in terms of food,
money, or clothes, but rarely in terms of
health.

If we have not begun to cope with our
limitations, we may find ourselves wallow-
ing in the negativity of self-pity or anger.
We may become so entangled in these self-
defeating thoughts that we lose our ability
to grow and to see other real choices. Instead of raging at the unfairness of poor
health or limited mobility, we can "make
do" with the strength, time, ability, and
creativity we still have.

*I will use what I have and not bemoan what I
don't have.*

*The great and glorious masterpiece of
man is to know how to live to purpose.*
— *Montaigne*

When we undergo any crisis, it's quite
common for self-esteem to take a plunge.
If life seems to hand us one crisis after another, our feelings of self-worth may vary
from day to day. Once we get used to
the newest change (perhaps this time it
is diminished health) we begin to realize
that only we are capable of nurturing ourselves.

We can solve some of our problems by
setting new, more realistic goals, goals
that we can reach successfully. Then our
damaged self-esteem can start to become
whole once again.

*I am capable of taking better care of myself by
setting challenging goals and by doing things I
love to do.*

April 18

He who conceals his disease cannot expect to be cured.
— *Ethiopian Proverb*

We gain very little if we use our problems to hide from other people and the realities of life. Yet, at times, we may drift into this negative attitude even though a reclusive life is self-serving, not the least bit enjoyable, and unfair to the people who care about us.

One way to survive is to develop the confidence we need to face others. Our problems should not be the first impression people have of us, but that is all we present if we are hiding our real selves from them. We have so much to offer — and so much to gain — when we set ourselves out on center stage and actively get on with living.

I am capable of buoying myself up to face each new challenge by moving out of my hiding places.

The only courage that matters is the kind that gets you from one moment to the next.

— *Mignon McLaughlin*

Morning sounds and sights filter in through the bedroom window as we lie awake wondering, once again, if we can get started for the day. Oh, we think to ourselves, can I make these tired and weary bones and these sore and aching muscles do what I command them to do one more time?

We need strength to begin, to face each day, to start working our joints so we can face another day. A silent prayer may rush from our lips as we gather all our resources. We are extraordinarily strong people. Having a health problem makes us aware of a source of strength previously left untapped. We open ourselves to that strength — within ourselves, our doctors, our Higher Power. We rise and get on with our lives.

I have two gifts right now — this day and the strength to meet its challenges and demands.

April 20

My mind to me a kingdom is,
Such present joys therein I find
That it excels all other bliss
That earth affords or grows by kind.
— *Sir Edward Dyer*

Within the private confines of our thoughts, we can build castles or dream of solving all the problems of the world. At times, we may still daydream like children who envision themselves as heroes, builders, or saviors. We may still unconsciously look for drama and excitement.

Maturity gives us something that our youthful selves would never have understood — compromise. We don't have to see compromise as surrender. For us, it can mean action. When faced with the reality of dreams that can't be achieved, we can compromise by building new dreams that not only are as important as our original ones, but also offer success.

My dreams can still direct the course of my life.

*To know
That which lies before us in daily life,
Is the prime wisdom.*
                                        — John Milton

It isn't easy becoming an adult. We have to pay the dues as we go along the path of life. As long as we have had joy and suffering, we may as well learn to use our well-earned adult perspective. After all, look how hard we worked to get here!

Enjoyment is still there, free for the taking. All the intangibles we enjoyed before are still there — love, honor, trust. We alone can decide, as we sift through the happenings of our days, whether to call our lives wreckage or success, whether to create delight or sorrow. A change in circumstances or health doesn't mean the end of joyful living. Such changes will often help us to begin living our lives more wisely, with greater appreciation and understanding.

I will find and accept the gift of joyful living today.

April 22

As mature people we must learn not to love ourselves excessively nor to mistrust the universe morbidly.
— *Joshua Loth Liebman*

Each time we know success, large or small, we may tend to applaud ourselves. We have all seen small children clapping their hands together in glee at some small triumph. That is the spontaneity of human nature.

Even now that we are older, we may find it difficult not to praise ourselves in front of others each time we make some kind of gain. We learn we are applauded for those special times with which all people can identify — success on the job or when a new child or grandchild is born. Sometimes, however, our applause must be private — treasured by no one but ourselves — for we may be the only ones to realize how much we deserve it.

When I achieve success, in any aspect of my life, I will glow with inner pride.

To everything there is a season, and a time to every purpose under the heaven.

— *Ecclesiastes 3:1*

All times and places in our lives have meaning and value. Regardless of what we have done in the past, whether we are proud or ashamed of our past actions, the only time over which we have any control is now. If we have no sense of direction in life, if we have no daily power or purpose, we may wander aimlessly through this new time in our lives, unaware of where we are going.

The reality of our lives is this: our health has changed. We are the only ones who can choose how to deal with this reality. We can wistfully look back to another time and place, or we can live in the here and now by making the best of a less than ideal situation. The choice is ours, but only the second choice provides our lives with meaning and purpose.

I won't squander today by living in the past.

April 24

To struggle when hope is banished.
To live when life's salt is gone!
To dwell in a dream that's
vanished —
To endure, and go calmly on!
— Ben Jonson

At times we all dwell in the mansions created by our own dreams. When dream rooms are the only ones we visit, however, reality will jar us back to the present. We then have only two choices: to move forward or to live continually in the past.

Just when it seems there is no future, that there is no chance to ever live a normal life again, a thread of hope surfaces, and we struggle onward. Recognition that we can — and are — still enduring gives rise to hope and helps us go calmly on.

Dreams are sacred to me, but I must live in the present so I can survive day to day.

*Every tub must stand on its own
bottom.*

— *Thomas Fuller*

As we accomplish each goal in our lives, we feel a tremendous sense of pride. Whether from success at the job, in school, or in a volunteer capacity, achieving a goal is personally gratifying.

The challenge that chronic illness presents is to reorganize our goals so they are still practical and attainable. If we spend our time complaining rather than changing, we may never learn to live successfully with the illness. It's not going to go away. Things will never be the same as before. Accepting this fact is a colossal challenge.

My faith in myself has waned with the onset of my illness. I am just realizing that I can still depend upon myself.

April 26

Kindness can become its own motive.
We are made kind by being kind.
— *Eric Hoffer*

Our own simple words to others can brighten our day. Too often we are caught up in the personal miseries of our lives, too involved to reach out to other people. We may forget that other people have the same needs we do. So many times, because we are ill or old or hurting, we expect others to come to us. That's not fair to them, and it's not good for us.

Kind words and actions toward others can help us through the hard times. We can smile at the elderly man all alone in the grocery check-out line. We can talk to neighbors, thank the young man who courteously holds a door open, and reach out in dozens of other ways to the people who even briefly touch our lives. It's good for them — and for us.

I will make an extra effort to reach out in kindness to my neighbors and friends.

Solitude: A good place to visit, but a poor place to stay.

— *Joan Billings*

We probably recognize our need for solitude in our lives — private time when we can sit and think, or listen to music, or simply enjoy the quiet. When solitude becomes a way of life, however, it can lead to loneliness, and loneliness can lead to self-pity. This is a dangerous position.

We tread a real tightrope with our need for solitude. We need to be alone, but not isolated. In our solitude, we can find serenity through meditation and prayer. Once we are reenergized, it will be easier for us to balance our lives by inviting a friend into our home or reaching out to another who is in pain. Solitude encourages us to turn our backs on loneliness and to reach out to others once again.

I will not impose a sentence of solitary confinement upon myself. I am still a valuable member of society.

April 28

Where there's music, there can be no evil.

— Cervantes

So many of us spent part of our childhoods glued to the radio, ears alert for our favorite stories and songs. Listening to music filled large parts of our days. The joy of music need not ever dim.

We can let the song within our heart burst forth, unbidden, to warm the memories of our souls and the texture of our days. Bubbling to the surface of awareness, music can create a twinkle in the eyes and cause a smile to burst into full bloom even on the shiest person's face.

We can use the magic of music to uplift a bad mood or dissipate our sadness. While listening to music, we can, for a while, forget our problems. Loving music is a special source of happiness we can carry with us wherever we go.

My warmest feelings can surface as I listen to or play music, and I can feel perfectly happy.

*You grow up the day you have the
first real laugh — at yourself.*
            — Ethel Barrymore

If we are always serious and never see
the funny side of life, there will be no
respite from our illness. It takes fewer
muscles to laugh than to cry. We'll
breathe easier and deeper, and we'll be
much more content when we laugh.

We can choose to pay attention to why
other people are laughing and learn to
laugh along with them. We can try every
day — even every hour — to find the positive or humorous side of life, for laughter
helps us put things into perspective. It
lends hope and meaning to life.

*I will open my eyes to the funny side of life and
laugh with others.*

April 30

Although the world is full of suffering,
it is also full of the overcoming of it.
— Helen Keller

It's easy to become overwhelmed with the day-to-day pain and annoyance of a chronic medical condition. We try hard, but every now and again our perspective gets knocked off center. We may begin to think only in terms of sickness and pain.

Sometimes it's difficult to find a kind thought or a warm spot for ourselves. If we shadow our lives with pain, frustration, and scorn, we will not be able to relax within the quiet confines of our days. Each day is new and fresh, and it's up to us to welcome it with joy and gratitude. It's up to us to overcome the obstacles to our happiness.

Today, I take the responsibility for my own happiness.

May

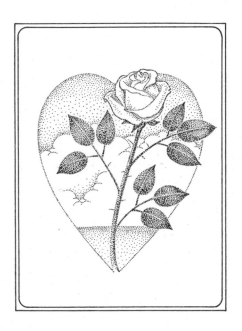

Blossoms are scattered by the wind and the wind cares nothing, but the blossoms of the heart no wind can touch.

— *Yoshida Kenko*

Our personal, private, or spiritual emotions are like unfolded blossoms within us. There, too, are other, less private emotions. The love and caring we harbor for those people who are closest to us are full-blooming flowers which give us everlasting joy.

While we may not react with any emotion to blossoms blowing in the wind, we may find ourselves ever awed as those very blossoms start as buds and then bloom within a summer season. The wonders of nature are like miracles — so are the wonders of humankind.

My innermost emotions blossom and grow within me and bear the fruit of maturity and love for others.

May 2

> *Wisdom denotes the pursuing of the*
> *best ends by the best means.*
> — *Francis Hutcheson*

Remember when we were youngsters and used to say, ''When I grow up, I'm going to . . .''? Somehow that magic moment never arrives. We grow a little each day, but change comes slowly.

We realize we have matured when we recognize our days as a series of options. Diminished health may change those options somewhat, but we still have choices to make.

We do not have a choice over the state of our health, but we can ''grow into'' acceptance and into more positive attitudes. We can achieve the best for ourselves.

Although some of my choices will be different from those I had originally planned, I can choose the best that life has to offer me now.

*In our own secret hearts we each
and all of us feel superior to the rest
of the world, or, if not superior, at
least "different" with a difference
that is very precious and beautiful to
us, and the base of all our pride and
perseverance.*

— *Solomon Eagle*

How alike we all are, yet how different.
Differences are what make each person so
special. All our efforts and all our experiences can shine forth ready to enhance
our lives and the lives of others when we
dare to let our differences show.

In this complex world, each of us and
our differences are needed. To find where
our uniqueness is most useful, we may
have to go out of our way. We may need
to actually create a niche for ourselves as
we have done so many times before. In
doing this, we affirm our value and that
of all others.

*I accept my differentness as a gift and a strength,
not a weakness.*

May 4

> *. . . I was the breadwinner.*
> *Only I didn't WIN the bread,*
> *I worked hard, and earned it. . . .*
> — *Elise Maclay*

When poor health slightly alters the way we live our lives, the adjustment is difficult but feasible. But when poor health alters the way we live our lives and wrenches away even our financial livelihood, the adjustment is far more difficult.

Sufferers of chronic medical conditions often must discontinue working and may have to depend upon loved ones or disability payments for income. It may take some time to regain perspective, to realize that whether we are working or not, we still have personal worth. What matters most is what kind of person we are, not what job we do.

Life has handed me a portion I did not choose and do not welcome, but I can choose my own response.

Learn to like what you are, for you take yourself with you wherever you go.

— *K. O'Brien*

A change in physical or mental health can lower our self-esteem. One of the hardest tasks we have to face is learning to accept who we are right now, not what we wanted to be.

Every day we have the right to assure ourselves that we are doing the very best job that we can do. Acceptance of ourselves allows us a serenity we've not known before. This doesn't mean giving up; in fact, it provides a base from which we can grow. Accepting where we are and who we are today gives us the honesty to admit our deficits. It gives us the confidence to really move forward. We can be proud that we are succeeding, even with this new and unwanted burden.

My illness has not changed who I am. The course of my life has been changed, but my direction remains the same — forward.

May 6

Troubles, like babies, grow larger by nursing.

— Lady Holland

The more we allow ourselves to fret about our troubles, the larger they appear to grow. Soon they are blown out of proportion.

Perhaps we need to set some time aside each day specifically for worrying. It's much easier to put our worrisome thoughts out of our minds if we know that we will deal with them at a certain time every day. This "worry time" will also give us the chance to decide whether we have any control over these problems or whether we should just let them go. None of us is without problems, and if we address them with some serious thinking time each day, we should be able to free our minds for some of the more important things in our lives — like personal growth and development of values.

I will strike a happy balance between worries and joys.

*Faith has a powerful effect in help-
ing people recover a sense of balance,
tranquility, and hope.*
                            — *Robert Veninga*

It's the funniest thing about human nature: When we are well we accept our
Higher Power with few second thoughts.
When we have undergone some kind of
crisis, however, large numbers of people
seem to lose their faith for a while. After
all, who among us hasn't asked, ''Why
me?'' when our health first took a turn
for the worse? Questioning our faith is
common at such a time.

A health crisis often encourages soul-
searching, and spiritual exploration. Life
as we knew it has gone topsy-turvy, and
we need time to adjust. After a while many
of us return with renewed strength to our
spiritual beliefs.

*My belief in my Higher Power may have dimin-
ished for a while, but I take comfort in knowing
that belief is always there.*

May 8

Leisure is the most challenging responsibility a man can be offered.
— *William Russell*

We are a work-oriented society. As children, we were taught to do our homework and the chores. We may have ''played house'' or pretended we were ''going to work.''

Play, therefore, can be a real challenge, especially for adults. Keyed up from a day in the work force or a day coping with the rigors of illness or pain, we can hardly settle down when busy thoughts crowd our consciousness. Leisure time can be a burden to us if we don't know how to creatively fill it.

Regardless of what our job is, at home or away, we can learn to set it aside when work is over. Playtime should become sacred, for it's a special time when we feed our need to be carefree and spontaneous.

Using my leisure time for play will keep me healthier, mentally and physically.

*The dark, uneasy world of family life
— where the greatest can fail and the
humblest succeed.*
                          — Randall Jarrell

We carry so much emotional baggage
from childhood into our adult lives. The
sum total of all our experiences forms our
personalities and, in the very essence of
our being, our spiritual selves. Less often
do the wonderful memories, the happier
times, spring forward in our minds. The
bad feelings, the sad memories, the hard
times — these are what we may remember
the most.

Who we came from, what we came
from, shouldn't define all that we can be
as adults. There may come a time when
regardless of our past experiences, we can
acknowledge them, put them aside, and
move on with our lives.

*I can put aside my past by facing my future with
hope and promise. I am looking for progress, not
perfection.*

May 10

Life would be infinitely happier if we
could only be born at the age of eighty
and gradually approach eighteen.
— Mark Twain

It isn't until we add many years to our
lives that we realize just how good most
of us had it at eighteen. We were, by
and large, only responsible for ourselves.
Hindsight is always twenty-twenty.

How nice for us that the hindsight we
have developed over the years can be used
to our benefit now. We understand that
it's natural for older people to lead and to
teach the younger ones. Paying for life's
experiences — joys and sorrows — hasn't
all been easy. We have earned the wisdom
we have now.

Since I could not be wise when I was young, the
wisdom I have gained with maturity will serve
me well as I get older.

*The emotions may be endless. The
more we express them, the more we
may have to express.*
— *E. M. Forster*

Like layers of paint, our resistance to
expressing our emotions can be peeled
away. Poor health may make us feel as
though we don't want to expend the effort
anymore. We may have withdrawn within
ourselves, isolated our feelings from risk
or hurt or disappointment.

Right now might be a good time to take
a long, hard look at ourselves. Are we
protecting ourselves by not discussing our
feelings or sharing our emotions with others? Not until those outer layers of fear,
loneliness, and pain are stripped away can
we get in touch with our emotions. Sur-
prising as it seems, when we let go of our
feelings and start to be totally honest with
ourselves, we find greater and deeper and
lovelier emotions to express.

*I can openly express my feelings to those closest
to me.*

May 12

Every day cannot be a feast of lanterns.

— *Chinese Proverb*

Many of us sometimes feel as though our lives are boring, as though each day is too predictable and routine. I'm missing something, we may think to ourselves, or there has to be more to life than this.

It's those times that we can remind ourselves to think of life as a journey. As with any lengthy trip, this one, too, has days in which the scenery is monotonous and uninspiring. But we're moving; we're making progress in our personal growth, and our attitudes are improving. Routine is not a bad thing, and it can be a good element of our lives when it gives form and balance to our days. Routine is often what gives us the time and energy to tackle new projects or to make changes.

Today, I will enjoy the calmness of my life. Within this calmness, I will dream and make plans for making my life even fuller.

Patience and fortitude conquer all things.
— *Ralph Waldo Emerson*

Remember how, as children, we waited for special occasions like birthdays and holidays? The waiting seemed endless. Adults would admonish us, "Have patience. Everything comes to those who wait."

We were always more than surprised when time seemed to pass more quickly by staying busy, just as our parents had said it would. As adults, we hear that in many instances the only way to conquer a problem is to wait it out. We can do nothing else, for no matter how important the awaited event or the news is, we can no more shorten the time than we could wish a speedy arrival of our birthdays when we were young. Now, as then, our only options are to have patience and to stay busy.

Now that I am not as well as before I am learning the true value of patience.

May 14

*A true friend is the most precious of
all possessions and the one we take the
least thought about acquiring.*
— La Rouchefoucauld

Even with honorable intentions we may,
once in a while, treat those who care about
us with less respect than they deserve.
When a chronic illness has entered our life
we can become obsessed with ourselves. It
is difficult to be anything but self-centered
at first because we are frightened and uncertain about the future.

It is then that we may alienate our closest friends with a boring daily litany of
symptoms. Gradually we learn that illness is only one part of our lives and that
dwelling on it serves no purpose and may
damage our friendships. When our obses-
sion with illness subsides, we become able
once again to express concern and interest
in others — the foundation of friendship.

*My friendships are invaluable. I will let my
friends know how much I cherish them.*

*Nothing has a stronger influence psy-
chologically on their environment,
and especially on their children, than
the unlived lives of the parents.*
— *Carl Jung*

Sometimes chronic illness emphasizes
flaws in our relationships. For whatever
reason — greater honesty, less tolerance,
or an increased need for openness — we
struggle more often with conflicting feelings toward our loved ones, especially our
parents.

It can be healing for us to review our
childhood years without blaming or em-
bellishment. We can look back and realize that our parents, too, were influenced
by their childhood years. Did they receive
the nurturing they needed? The love they
deserved? Thinking about our parents in
this way reminds us to live with forgiveness for ourselves and for everyone whose
lives we touch.

*I will allow myself to look back on my parents
with forgiveness.*

May 16

Life is a series of experiences, each one of which makes us bigger, even though it is hard to realize this.
— Henry Ford

During these most devastating periods of our lives, it is hard to recognize that we will, in the long run, benefit from the experience. As we live through painful or trying times when we are barely surviving, we certainly are not aware of growing or of learning something.

Yet, in the more quiet times of our lives, when we're not in pain or just hanging on by a thread, we can see that, yes, I did learn this or, indeed, that event did force me to grow. Chronic illness is no different from other crises, and we are able to inventory ourselves and see healthier attitudes and stronger character as results of what we've experienced.

I will take time today to list the ways in which some ''bad'' experiences have helped me become a better or more mature person.

When you dig another out of trouble,
you find a place to bury your own.
> — *Anonymous*

When acting the way people expect us to, we may help others, but does it really come from the heart? Frequently people act not out of compassion or caring, but because that's how they feel others will expect them to behave.

When helping others in a completely unselfish manner, we need no kudos from anyone, for we have no ulterior motive other than helpfulness. Willingness to assist other people with their problems creates some freedom from our own.

I will know I have become less selfish when I don't have a moment's hesitation before helping another human being.

May 18

Pain is part of being alive, and we need to learn that. Pain does not last forever, nor is it necessarily unbearable, and we need to be taught that.
— *Harold Kushner*

Losing anything — a loved one, a favorite book, even a set of goals we thought were reachable — can hurt deeply. But the loss of good health is one of the greatest pains we can suffer, for it signifies the ending of what is familiar and what is expected. The pain of a long-term medical condition isn't just physical, it's also emotional. We are afraid that we will not be able to live through the change.

With time, however, we adjust to this latest loss, just as we have adjusted to others. We create new routines that allow for diminished health. As laughter filters through our days once again, we understand that even despair is not permanent.

I reach outward, extending my arms for hope. I turn inward with the thought of helping myself. I am getting stronger.

*The thought of suicide is a great con-
solation: by means of it one gets successfully through many a bad night.*
— *Friedrich Wilhelm Nietzsche*

Many of us pretend that the thought
of suicide has never crossed our minds,
but our thoughts may occasionally become
morbid — and we may be frightened.

These thoughts may seem harmful, but
they may actually be helpful. Thoughts
of suicide can force us to recognize how
much we value living.

As we contemplate the moment at which
our life would end, we struggle and notice our desire for life, although we may
not understand why we have this desire.
What's important is that we gave ourselves
the choice of death and did not choose it.
As we feel the joy of that decision we can
think more of ourselves and of our worth.
We really do want to live and are strong
enough to know that suicide is not an acceptable solution to our problems.

I feel joy from knowing I can choose life.

May 20

Stripped of all their masquerades, the fears of men are quite identical: the fear of loneliness, rejection, inferiority, unmanageable anger, illness and death.

— *Joshua Loth Liebman*

Sometimes we may try to hold ourselves apart from others, pretending our uniqueness makes us superior. Underneath all our bluff and bravado we recognize that our fears are shared by all people.

We fashion our lives to protect ourselves from hurt, from displeasing those we love, and from disappointing ourselves. Our best chance for success, despite some difficult burdens, is to develop a positive attitude, an open nature, and a willingness to risk. Doing this doesn't necessarily protect us from all our fears, but it does create an honest bond with other people who also accept their human nature.

My fears don't have to isolate me; in fact, they can be the means by which I reach out to others.

Out of a sense of duty and a desire to protect a loved one, a vicious cycle of misinterpretation, guesswork, silence, and isolation is initiated.
— Neil A. Fiore

For a while we may have tried to protect our loved ones by not talking about our illness. We may have even secretly hoped that it would go away if we didn't talk about it. We learned, however, that this would never be and that problems often escalate if they are not dealt with.

We see more clearly now that we can't protect our family members or our friends. Trying to protect them meant denying our own feelings and ignoring theirs. We've discovered that our loved ones don't need to be — and often don't want to be — protected. And when we don't protect them, we've found that we and the people we love are growing and becoming stronger.

I can be honest with my loved ones about my feelings and needs.

May 22

> *Happiness is like time and space —*
> *we make and measure it ourselves; it*
> *is as fancy, as big, as little, as you*
> *please; just a thing of contrasts and*
> *comparisons.*
>
> — *George du Marier*

Happiness is a reference point, a relative state of mind to which we compare other emotions. Being happy is one of our ultimate goals. How we get there or if we get there often depends on how we live and how we treat other people.

When we were children, many of our needs were taken care of by others. Now, it is more often we who must create our own happiness. We are no longer children dependent on others for our dreams and joys. We are adults, free to make our happiness in any form or shape we wish.

My happiness depends on me, not on others.

Prayer, crystallized in words, assigns
a permanent wave-length on which
the dialogue has to be continued.
— *Dag Hammarskjold*

Many of us have all but forgotten how to pray. We don't mean to avoid prayer — it just happens. Instead of prayer, we look to ourselves for answers or to others for our well-being. Our spiritual lives have become stagnant.

The reality of illness has, for many of us, underscored the limited power we have over some areas of our lives. We have no power over diagnoses, prognoses, remissions, or side-effects of medications. Whether out of anger, pain, depression, or hopelessness, a need arises to find balance in a world suddenly gone crazy. We may then turn to a Power greater than ourselves to provide the comfort we so desperately need. We pray; we meditate. We find peace.

I don't have to carry my burdens alone.

May 24

*Whatever you may be sure of, be sure
of this — that you are dreadfully like
other people.*
— *James Russell Lowell*

Scientists have long known that all human bodies have essentially the same structure. In this day and age, one person's heart — or even other organs — can be implanted into another human being's body.

Other similarities come to mind as we live the day-by-day struggles of having a long-term medical condition. We share the frustrations, the unshed tears, pain, and hopelessness with all people whose state of health is forever altered. But we also share in joy, in pleasure, in the small and large successes we all can achieve as we move on with our lives. We are different, but we are also so very much the same.

Despite my physical limitations, I am more like all other people than I am different from them. Today, I will look for those similarities.

Much of your pain is self-chosen. It is the bitter potion by which the physician within you heals your sick self.
— *Kahlil Gibran*

We rarely, if ever, think of grief in terms of loss of good health, yet each of us moves through the grieving process. We have a tendency to drive away those who are closest to us — those who are willing to share our pain — because we are unsure of how to handle our crisis.

The period of time in which we grieve leaves us emotionally raw, open, and vulnerable. We may refuse help because of stubborn pride, totally unaware that the people who care about us are in pain and need to share as well. Fortunately grief passes, and while we will never be the same, we do heal.

Loss of good health is new to me, and I must learn how to be gracious to those who care about me.

May 26

> *Know the true value of time; snatch,*
> *seize, and enjoy every moment of it.*
> *No idleness, no laziness, no procras-*
> *tination, never put off till tomorrow*
> *what you can do today.*
> — *Lord Chesterfield*

Whether the memories were good or bad, we can never call back those moments that are already gone. Each special time should be savored as unique, never to be repeated again.

We may be uncertain of what our future holds, especially since we are not as well as before. By understanding the preciousness of each day, we can enhance the way we live our lives.

Each day is valuable and offers us one-time opportunities to seize that moment — to make the very most of each chance to live.

Every moment is precious. I will make the most of each day.

*True miracles are created by men
where they use the courage and intelligence that God gave them.*
— *Jean Anouilh*

Recently a woman in Minnesota received her Ph.D. She was eighty years
old. She said she needed to conquer new
worlds.

The quest for learning should never
end, yet all too often we feel our education ends when we are done with school.
If we want something intensely enough,
whether we set our sights for an education or some other goal, it's very likely
we will find a way of achieving our needs.
Sometimes in the process of getting there,
we discover other tracks to follow, which
may take us to a slightly different endpoint
than the one we had originally envisioned.
We learn, as mature adults, to accept sub-
stitutes. And still we reach as far as we
are able.

*I can learn to set new goals — ones which
challenge me but don't defeat me.*

> *Very few live by choice. Every man is placed in his present condition by causes which acted without his foresight, and with which he did not always willingly operate.*
> — *Samuel Johnson*

How does a person cope with a chronic illness? Our lives are formed by the events around us; these events often move forward of their own volition, without our permission or even our willingness. Now that the problem is obvious, living with that change will test our characters.

Those of us who have learned to cope with radically altered lifestyles and who can still love, laugh, and cry are survivors. We may not like our portion in life, but we are determined to handle it well.

I haven't chosen all the changes in my life, but I can choose to accept the changes and to live a warm and sharing life.

*There is a period of life when we
swallow a knowledge of ourselves and
it becomes either good or sour inside.*
— *Pearl Bailey*

We have a tendency to hold on to those
dreams, goals, and images we had when
we were young. When we accept the
reality of what our lives have become —
good or bad — we are finally adult.

It's far easier to accept external realities
than our deeper, more personal internal
realities. Accepting that we are never
going to be tall or agile or rich is simpler
than admitting that we are selfish or angry
or unkind. Perhaps the external things are
easier because there is nothing we can do
to change them, and we resist admitting
to character defects because those can be
changed. We may not like what we see,
but if we swallow that bitter pill we are
able to change.

*I will ignore my fear and admit to the good and
bad within me. This gives me the freedom to
change.*

I expect to pass through life but once. If, therefore, there can be any kindness I can show, or any good thing I can do to any fellow human being, let me do it now.

— *William Penn*

Each night, as we place our heads upon our pillows, we can think back over the day and remember the things we said or did that added pleasure to others' lives. Usually, those same words and actions add joy to our lives too.

During our lives we have passed by multiple opportunities to be kind to others — there are no second chances. But what we can do is be aware of those special opportunities now and make the very best of them.

My new awareness of life's fleeting opportunities will help me show my kinder side more often.

Laughter is a tranquilizer with no side effects.

— *Arnold Glasow*

Good friends laughing together can warm the heart of even a casual onlooker. Unlike medicine, laughter costs us nothing and can be partaken of as often as we see fit.

When illness clouds our lives, it's nice to know that one thing stays the same — we can still laugh. At ourselves. With friends. At a funny television program.

A good hearty laugh is therapy for our minds and bodies. Mirthful laughter can cause a remarkable feeling of well-being and joy. Laughter loosens all the cares and woes of the day and makes them somehow easier to bear.

Laughing openly and spontaneously will always make me feel better.

June

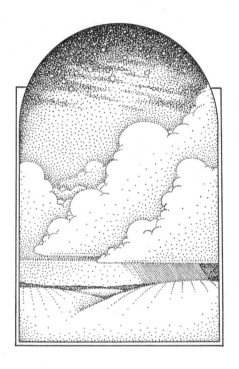

*Sorrows are like thunderclouds — in
the distance they look black; over our
heads scarcely gray.*
                    — Jean Paul Richter

We sometimes become consumed by
worry over things we think we need to do
or decide or complete. Often, this concern
is caused by us — not our problems —
because we're trying to solve all problems
and make all decisons at once.

Seen as whole, all the events in a lifetime can be overwhelming. Our fears, our
sorrows, our anguish over the loss of good
health, the loss of time, or even the loss
of someone we loved very much, can be
completely consuming. Yet if we learn to
take our sorrows one by one, to dissect
them into little pieces, we find that we
can accept our sorrows as only a part of
our lives. We still can endure. Taken one
at a time, our sorrows will dissipate into
wispy, insubstantial clouds.

*All things are manageable when I see them as a
series of small items.*

June 2

All our reasoning ends in surrender to feeling.
— Blaise Pascal

In all our endeavors it is apparent that success is possible only with persistent effort. We must all pay the price to achieve any worthwhile goal. We shouldn't be surprised when negative thoughts enter our minds. These thoughts do not go away easily. We have human frailties, so our thoughts are often disorganized and feelings are too subdued or excessive. Perfection is not possible no matter how hard we try. But we can search for answers.

We can't have things both ways, so we have to make choices. We can think through the trade-off before we make a choice. Whatever our choice, we should make it and accept it. Squandered chances to solve problems may be lost forever.

I struggle with the same problems over and over again. Today, I resolve to start my search to find some answers.

There are no gains without pain.
— *Adlai Stevenson*

Parents often are surprised that their children seem to change before their very eyes. The same is true in how we deal with each day. It was frightening when we experienced the toppling of many parts of our lives which had given us comfort and which we had expected to continue to comfort us. We may have initially thought that we'd never be able to reconstruct a productive life.

But we have been able to rebuild our lives. Like toddlers, we have taken a few small steps forward each day. Day after day, we've strengthened ourselves by making steady, but small, advances. Step by step we've re-created our lives, often without recognizing our growth. Then, suddenly, we look at our lives, and we are amazed at how far we've come. Amazed — and proud.

Today, I will take time to measure my growth, both emotionally and spiritually.

June 4

*The supreme happiness of life is the
conviction that we are loved.*
— *Shakespeare*

Unqualified love is the assurance that,
regardless of how we look or act or live,
we will be loved. We don't have to earn
it; we don't have to measure up to it.
Many of us were lucky enough to have
been loved in this way by our parents and
other family members. We were hugged,
we were accepted — no matter what.

Some of us weren't that lucky; we may
spend a large part of our adult lives looking for that love. Fortunately, we've
learned that we don't have to find it; we
only have to give it — we can love ourselves in a totally unqualified manner. We
can't change the events of the past, but we
can change the influence of those events
on the present.

*The feeling of loving myself and being loved by
others warms and nurtures my life.*

*I make myself laugh at everything, for
fear of having to weep.*
— *Beaumarchais*

Sometimes we may want to cry. We
might even feel within our eyes the burn-
ing of tears about to come, but we don't
allow them to come. Perhaps we blink
them back or avert our eyes so that others won't see. After all, we may reason,
someone might see and want to give us
undue attention or — worse yet — pity.

As we deal with our emotions, there
are two issues involved — acknowledging
our emotions and showing them. We may
choose not to show all our emotions to
others, but we do want to recognize them
ourselves. Denying our negative emotions
is counterproductive to the honesty we
need as we build a full life. We can give
ourselves permission to feel sad as well as
joyous, to be angry as well as happy. They
are honest feelings.

*I am at the beginning of a journey to discover
my emotions.*

June 6

*Prayer is not asking. It is a longing
of the soul.*
— *Mohandas Gandhi*

Some people have suggested that we
shouldn't ask for something in prayer. Yet
our need to pray is often fueled by emotional or physical pain or by confusion or
doubt. Certainly we can't — certainly we
shouldn't — wait for distressing situations
to pass before we pray or meditate.

Our souls long for balance and serenity,
and we find this when we turn our pain,
doubts, and fears over to the comforting
presence of our Higher Power. Often what
we seek is not an answer to a question
as much as a sense of being loved and
understood. When we can't find these
in our physical world, we reach out with
our spiritual selves to a balancing presence
that understands our deepest pains and
fears and our greatest joys.

*No matter what I express in prayer, I am com-
forted in knowing I'm understood.*

To know how to grow old is the master-work of wisdom, and one of the most difficult chapters in the great art of living.
— *Henri Frederic Amiel*

We often strive to imitate people we admire — special teachers, our parents, or friends. Many older people we choose to emulate have remained productive members of their communities and have found significant ways to help people. If we can be active, busy, and helpful we will not only enhance our lives, we become the role models for those younger than we are.

There are some people who seem to age so gracefully that they have the ability to make everyone around them feel special. We all appreciate friends like that, and we can become that way too.

I will live my life so well that I am a role model for young people.

June 8

Sometimes what we think is so impossible turns out to be possible after all.

— *K. O'Brien*

The pure joy of imagination is that it holds no bounds. Even if we are tethered by poor health we can still believe there are better days ahead. And in truth, we can find worthwhile ways to spend our precious time and energy if we wish.

Time spent lost in thought is not wasted, for these precious moments let us remember wonderful times gone by and allow us to rehearse our role in the future. We should imagine ourselves as proud and fully capable. This may, of course, not be true, but the more we try the better we will be able to present ourselves in public. The easier it is for us to be in public, the more often we will go out.

I am not wasting time when I daydream, for my dreams help me accept the changes in my life and allow me to practice for the future.

No man is an island, entire of itself.
　　　　　— *John Donne*

It's sometimes easy to develop a sense of aloneness. During our emotional and physical lows, we might sadly or bitterly isolate from other people because we feel so different from them. Our lives seem so much more complicated than theirs.

Usually, though, we do not choose to be completely independent of others. As we go through the motions of our day, our lives are touched by many people. They are part of the normal rhythm and flow of our experience.

And we are part of theirs. In hundreds of ways, we all support and nurture each other. We share their joys and pains because we care, because we're human.

When I am in need, caring people surround me. I will make sure that I am available for others when they need me too.

June 10

Pain is hard to bear. . . .
But with patience, day by day,
Even this shall pass away.
— *Theodore Tilton*

When emotional or physical pain becomes unbearable, the duration of each day seems longer than twenty-four hours. Any movement is intolerable; any attempt to begin the day is met with the shrilling objections of the voice of pain.

It is at this exact moment, each time it occurs, that we are tempted to give up the fight and become invalids. Then something prods us to try just one more time — just one more day. And so we struggle, and we are amazed to discover that we have successfully met and conquered another sunrise and another sunset. The strength to go on was there all the time, deep within us.

When my pain becomes greater than I can ever remember, I must draw on my inner resources to keep going.

*What we call the beginning is often
the end. And to make an end is to
make a beginning. The end is where
we start from.*

— *George Eliot*

Sometimes a painful ending can be the
beginning of a new way of life which is
a happy reality. The end of grief brings
us new acceptance and balance. The end
of a bad relationship might be a welcome
beginning.

An ending? Or a beginning? Often the
answer depends on how we choose to see
it. Grown children leaving home can be
a sad end, or it can be an exciting opportunity to begin living more for ourselves.
A move can mean leaving old friends or
meeting new ones. Almost every event in
life — marriage, a new job, graduation,
even a vacation — means an ending of
some sort. As we face each ending, we
can choose to see a new beginning.

*Today, I will remember that life is made of many
new beginnings.*

June 12

Develop an expanding sense of wonder at the world, at yourself, at God. The world will never starve for wonders — only for the want of wonder.
— *Bernard S. Raskas*

A crisis in our lives can make us cruel and bitter but can also cause us to do some soul-searching. Those of us who take inventory, who soul-search, may have a personal awakening to our capacity for joy and giving. Being aware of the beauty and symmetry that constantly surround us allows the horizons of our minds to expand.

As our sense of spirituality becomes whole again, we are aware of our impact upon others and upon nature.

A spiritual sense of self is important in my quest to find out who I am and what kind of person I want to be.

A desperate disease requires a danger-ous remedy.
— *Guy Fawkes*

Safety is important to all of us, but sometimes it is so important that we refuse to take risks. We may stay in unhealthy relationships or ignore our own or others' bizarre behavior because we're afraid of leaving the safety of our routine.

We become more willing, however, to take risks when things become desperate. Then we might take desperate measures. We might seek counseling or file for divorce in order to rescue or end a hurting relationship. If we feel emotionally upset, we might ask for professional help. That, too, involves taking a risk. These decisions don't come lightly. There is much soul-searching involved but we're able to make the decision when we realize that safety is sometimes more dangerous than risk.

I can make choices that are good for me, even if they threaten my safe routine.

June 14

Do not sit long with a sad friend,
When you go to a garden,
do you look at the flowers?
Spend more time with roses and
jasmines.

— *Jelaluddin Rumi*

Sometimes we slip over the boundary line of a close friendship. Up to that point, it may have been a real union, a true meeting of the minds. But then we might not only share our thoughts and our problems, but take on each other's problems as if they were our own. We may become obsessed with finding answers for our friends.

Just as we don't focus on the weeds in our garden, we can't see only the negative aspects of our friends' lives. We can be supportive, but we serve our friends and ourselves best when we let them confront their own problems.

I will remember that friends can comfort each other, but cannot carry the other's burdens.

Not the power to remember, but the power to forget is a necessary condition for our existence.

— *Sholem Asch*

To live happily in a relationship we cannot repeatedly dredge up the past, using it as a brickbat to pound another human being into submission. Yet we all have a tendency to do just that. ''I told you so,'' and ''You should have listened when I gave you advice,'' and ''You were wrong'' are phrases we may catch ourselves uttering.

We can learn to give up that final piece of control, that part which attempts to manipulate another human being with guilt. We can't change another human being. Our willingness to forgive errors, large and small, will mark our own personal growth. Forgiveness is in our own self-interest; we aren't free until we forgive.

Today, I will let go of one grudge. As I grow in understanding, I will grow in forgiveness.

June 16

We do not live an equal life, but one of contrasts and patchwork; now a little joy, then a sorrow, now a sin, then a generous or brave action.
— *Ralph Waldo Emerson*

As our life experience unfolds, we live some days to the fullest and others in a very minimal way. If we focus too much on the less productive days or if we use them only as substandard comparisons to our best days, we may lose sight of the real value and meaning of the time we've been given.

A wholesome life, a productive life, a good life — whatever we call it — is not a shimmering length of perfectly woven cloth. It's more like a patchwork quilt set together by resourceful hands. We cannot choose to discard a bad experience or a poor decision; instead, we piece it into the total colorful work that is life.

Today, I will be more aware of how the contrasts of my life create a unique and beautiful pattern.

Variety is the mother of enjoyment.
— *Benjamin Disraeli*

Ideally, we anticipate awakening in the morning, not sure what the day is going to bring, but looking forward to it anyway. Sometimes this eagerness comes more easily, for we have places to go and people to see. At other times, we're unable to recapture our previous joy. What took away our excitement for life? What can we do to reclaim it?

Life does not end at retirement or when the children move away or when our good health is diminished. It just changes. We can develop some new interests and hobbies. We can reexamine old attitudes and come up with new perspectives. Music and good fellowship with others can enrich our lives and strengthen us to go on. We can turn to our spiritual natures, and we will know joy.

I am aware of the wonders and opportunities around me. I will share the joy I find.

June 18

Never believe in faith, see for yourself!
What you yourself don't learn, you
don't know.
— *Bertolt Brecht*

While faith seems to be the watchword here, this quotation also extols the value of learning. Learning is not the opposite of faith. In fact, it supports and builds our faith. We often can trust our intuitions to guide us through all the lessons life provides us. It's up to us to pick and choose, to decide what lessons would be particularly pertinent to us, and to incorporate that knowledge into our own spirituality.

We learn firsthand, of course, from our own day-to-day lessons in living, but we also learn from the experiences of others, and these are equally beneficial to us. We can see for ourselves.

Learning strengthens my faith — in my Higher Power, in others, and in myself. I can use that greater faith to enhance and strengthen the quality of my life.

*We can either change the complexities
of life . . . or develop ways that enable
us to cope more effectively.*
— *Herbert Benson*

Our illnesses have brought many new complexities into our lives, and our reactions may become much more intense as time goes on — especially if we feel helpless or pity ourselves.

All people have crises in their lives. Our medical conditions don't give us immunity from the normal problems, pains, and disappointments that all of us must face. If anything, we may have an advantage over people who have never had health problems; we have learned some coping skills in dealing with our medical conditions. Also, we have become more open to advice and support from others. We can be proud of how far we've come; we can be optimistic of how far we can go.

I will gladly exchange help and support with my friends.

June 20

Be content to grow a little each day.
If the improvement is the sort of thing
which is very slow, do not measure it
too often. Do a self-comparison every
two weeks, or every six months —
whatever is appropriate.
                    — Lewis F. Presnall

It's not easy to change the way our
minds have been set, but sometimes we
really need to sit back and take stock of
how we have chosen to live — in both
large and small ways. We may realize
that we are racing about without so much
as a moment for our own well-being. We
might even delude ourselves that we enjoy
what we are doing so much that it is for
our well-being.

What matters most is that we vary the
pace of our days. We need the fast times,
but the slower, easier times are essential
for our total health — emotional, physical,
social, and spiritual.

I will slow down and spend some quiet time with
myself today.

*One cloud is enough to eclipse all the
sun.*

— *Thomas Fuller*

Sometimes a beautiful day suddenly
falls to pieces because of a criticism from
a friend or being stuck in traffic before
an important appointment. Later we may
have wondered why one small happening
could overshadow other happy events.

Quite possibly the answer lies within us
and our expectations. If we expect each
day and all our relationships to be without mishaps or misunderstandings, we set
ourselves up to be disappointed. If we
direct our energies toward pleasing our
friends and relatives at the expense of our
own needs and values, we are placing too
much responsibility in their hands. We
can have more rewarding days when our
expectations are realistic. Each day will
have unexpected delays or unappreciated
remarks, but they are just a scattering of
clouds in a bright, wide, wonderful sky.

I will have more realistic expectations.

June 22

*Disability usually puts a strain on a
good marriage and exposes a bad one.*
— *Robert Lovering*

The strain on relationships of chronically ill people is clearly shown in the fact
that their divorce rate is higher than the
national average. Perhaps this is not so
strange, since any stressful situation only
serves to point out any preexisting deficits.

Suffering is a personal and lonely state
even though others have been where we
are now. We can share some of our pain
with others. We can perhaps be an in-
spiration to them because of how well we
handle our suffering. We still can choose
our attitudes and our responses. Even
though there are some situations we cannot control, there is always hope and help.
We can receive relief and understanding.

*I will try to stay aware, in all my relationships,
of the added stresses caused by illness.*

*The degree and kind of sexuality of
a human being reaches up into the
ultimate pinnacle of his spirit.*
— *Friedrich Nietzsche*

Having a long-term medical problem
presents new problems, which we have
to cope with as part of our total picture.
One area that may present difficulties is
sexuality.

Sexuality is how we think about ourselves, of how we present ourselves, of all
that makes us unique. Our self-image may
bottom out as we undergo the daily rigors
of a medical problem, and we may for a
time feel unsexual and unsensual. It takes
us a while to realize that we still have the
same needs we always had — to be touched
and to feel good about ourselves. We don't
have to be silent or passive. We need love
and support, and sometimes we have to
ask before our needs can be met.

*I will remember that the quality of a relationship
depends on both people involved.*

June 24

> *There is a magnet in your heart that will attract true friends. That magnet is unselfishness, thinking of others first.*
>
> — *Paramahansa Yogananda*

Friendships develop slowly and are based on mutual interests and understanding. They are tested by time, by changes in life circumstances, and even by health. To be a real friend means being there when the chips are down, even when no one else is. It means giving and not receiving, but trusting that our friends are prepared to do the same.

Real friends take risks for one another — especially emotional risks — and still don't leave. A cherished friendship is not questioned, for we know, deep in our hearts, that we will always be there to help our close friends. We know they will always be there to help us.

I have strong and rewarding relationships. I cherish my friendships.

*Nothing is more fatal to health than
an overcare of it.*
— *Benjamin Franklin*

Let's face it. There are certain times
when we become preoccupied with our
health. After all, if we'd broken a leg we'd
be abnormal if we weren't concerned with
how we were going to walk or how frustrating it was. Long-term medical problems are a different matter. If we continue
to constantly talk about our health, we will
drive away the people we need most.

Talking less about our health problems
may have benefits. We won't be wear-
ing down our friends and family members
with our lengthy medical discussions, and
we also may become more accepting. To
be alive is to experience challenges, problems, and conflicts. Acceptance ensures
that we'll overcome some of the pain and
that hope will be renewed.

*Acceptance does bring relief and peace. God
will grant me the serenity to accept the things I
cannot change.*

June 26

A man can't retire his experience. He must use it.

— *Bernard Baruch*

We may want to pretend that some of our life experiences didn't happen to us, but they did happen. We even helped create some of our bad experiences. We are the sum total of all those experiences.

We can own our behaviors and attitudes and even admit to the ones we are not comfortable with. By doing so, we are not permanently passing judgment on ourselves. We can use our negative experiences as a basis for the changes we need to make. Our weaknesses can be useful to us when we let them teach us where we need to begin our change. They will lead us to new attitudes and strengths we will be proud to claim as our own. When we are ready, we can create and accept improvements in ourselves.

I am the sum total of all my experiences. I can use my past experiences to guide me into positive change.

*The sky is not less blue because the
blind man does not see it.*
       — *Danish Proverb*

Each day we make our choices anew.
We can choose to believe that pain and disappointment are the bitter fruits of living,
or we can trust in our ability to build harmony, enthusiasm, and gratefulness from
our day's experiences. We can hear the
music of children's voices at play or be irritated at the disruption. We can pray, or
we can chew on our anger.

We choose how we will see the world. If
we feel anger and despair, if we hear only
noise, if we see only dark, threatening
clouds — that is our reality. But our
negative choices don't change the world.
Birds' songs and children's voices still fill
the air. People still reach out to each other
through love and caring. And the bright
splash of sky is as blue as ever.

*Today, my reality will be based on the positive
things around me.*

June 28

Believe and remember this: every saint and every sinner affects those whom he will never see, because his words and deeds stamp themselves upon the soft clay of human nature everywhere.

— *Joshua Loth Liebman*

In a world of billions of people, it's easy to feel insignificant. As a result, we might excuse ourselves for not acting upon our sense of rightness. After all, we might reason, what difference does it make? At those times, we've forgotten about the ripple effect.

Occasionally we've even seen our words and actions rippling from one person to another, but more often we see nothing at all. Then we must choose — whether to bitterly reject the idea of making a difference or to trust that someone, somewhere, is being comforted by a ripple of the wave we dared to make.

My presence is felt by people I know — and by people I'll never know.

*Give thanks for sorrow that teaches
you pity; for pain that teaches you
courage — and give exceeding thanks
for the mystery which remains a mystery still — the veil that hides you
from the infinite, which makes it possible for you to believe in what you
cannot see.*

— *Robert Nathan*

We cannot run away from problems.
Tremendous problems — like a spouse
with a chronic illness — must be con-
fronted and resolved. Fears can be overwhelming. Tasks seem endless, and the
challenge seems too great. It is comforting to realize we face nothing alone.

We can't always be courageous, but fear
is dispelled by our inner strength, by our
trust that we will overcome problems and
do as well as is possible. We can talk to
ourselves in positive ways.

*I will not allow fear and panic to overtake me
today. Courage will open the door to wisdom
and peace of mind.*

June 30

> *The lame man who keeps the right road outstrips the runner who takes a wrong one. Nay, it is obvious that the more active and swift the latter is the further he will go astray.*
> — Francis Bacon

As we travel through life, distractions keep us from reaching our destination. Sometimes a wonderful, happy circumstance changes our direction, or a goal may be changed by the intrusion of a serious medical condition.

Regardless of altered courses, we want to keep our goals in sight. We must set goals which, whatever our circumstances, we know are attainable. To feel successful and proud of ourselves, we must be able to attain our new goals. And we can if we aim toward ideals that provide dreams, challenges, and the possibility of success.

I follow the path that is best for me and follow my own road map.

July

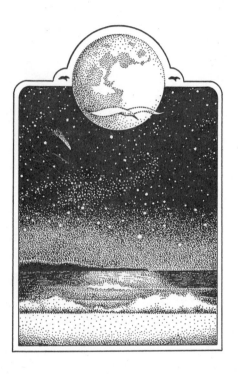

Time flies . . . Time has wings . . .
Time and tide wait for no man.
— *Proverbs*

We all have problems, but we deal with them in different ways. Some of us try to remove ourselves from the scene of our unhappiness. We get out of relationships, leave jobs, move away from our homes. Eventually, most of us realize that we have taken the major problems — ourselves and our behavior — with us. Time seems to crawl until we confront ourselves, decide to get help, and start to create change.

We need to make a true assessment of our problems. Then we can decide how willing we are to change those personal factors which contribute to the problems. Our load will begin to lighten, and time will once again have wings.

I recognize that my behavior dictates a large part of my life. I am responsible for my own actions.

July 2

If I'd known I was going to live so long, I'd have taken better care of myself.

— Leon Eldred

We had few concerns when we were young other than eating, sleeping, and playing with friends. As we grew into young adulthood, we worked hard and played hard, often ignoring any signals our bodies gave us. We expected to be stiff after exercise, for example, and accepted it as part of our lifestyle.

By the time our chronic medical conditions became evident, our health habits were fairly well-established. We certainly can't undo the early care — or neglect — of our bodies. But we can learn new habits that will serve us well all the days of our lives.

Ultimately, my physical and emotional health depends upon my willingness to take care of myself.

*A chronic illness is a constant and
sometimes overwhelming companion
. . . only the power of a warm heart
can alleviate the deep chill.*
— *Robert K. Massie*

When our lifestyles change and an illness pervades our lives, we often feel
lonely. It's not like a bad mood we can
just shake off.

We need our friends and family around
us, but it's up to us to give them the
cue. People may stay at arm's length until
we allow — even encourage — them to
come closer. We need the support they
can give us, and they need the satisfaction
of contributing to our lives no matter how
we've changed in our illness. We comfort
and encourage each other, and we all feel
blessed.

*My illness has not changed the basic person I
am. I needed the love and support of others
before. I still do.*

July 4

Judge a tree from its fruit; not from the leaves.

— *Euripides*

Sometimes we have a tendency to judge too quickly. Unfortunately, this is particularly true when we see people who are obviously physically impaired. We may form opinions of them based only on the fact that they walk differently or perhaps because they use a wheelchair.

We can judge people as individuals — not because of a medical condition. We can understand that people make their own individual marks on the world, not so much because of their physical abilities, but because of their mental and spiritual presence.

I will look beyond the external features of people and find the unique qualities within.

*When we do the best that we can, we
never know what miracle is wrought
in our life, or in the life of another!*
— *Helen Keller*

When we toss a pebble into a pond,
the widening concentric circles continue to
spread — the ripple effect — long after the
pebble is out of sight. Often the actions we
take have similar results.

We don't always know what effect our
lives and choices will have on other people. The immediate effects of our daily
lives are probably easier to gauge, but often we don't see the long-term effect we
have on others. And that really doesn't
matter because all we are urged to do is
to let kindness and responsibility rule our
decisions. The immediate effect we see is
the sense of growth within ourselves; the
long-term effect we can trust to be a miracle that we may never see.

*I'll remember that my actions affect many people
beyond me.*

July 6

Yesterday is a cancelled check; tomorrow is a promissory note; today is the only cash you have — so spend it wisely.

— Kay Lyons

Each day is a small fragment of a lifetime. This fact frees us to focus on the things we truly can influence. We can never return to the past, except within our memories. And we don't know what the future holds in store. The only time we can ''spend'' is today; the only time we touch is right now.

The simplicity of the present allows us to let go of the past and to ignore the unknowns of the future. Thus freed, we can set about the business of enriching our lives physically, emotionally, and spiritually. Unpleasant debts to the past are paid, and we've mortgaged nothing to the future. We are free to invest in growth by using the ''cash'' we have on hand.

This day is a valuable piece of my life. I will spend it well.

Smiles form the channels of a future tear.

— *Lord Byron*

We have often watched smiles turn to laughter and laughter back to tears. At a family reunion, we hear the joyous sounds of people chattering away, trying to catch up in five minutes for twenty lost years.

People who have Parkinson's disease sometimes complain that their faces don't match the emotions they want to express. The mask of the illness slows down normal movement of facial muscles. Even more tragic is the person who doesn't feel emotion. No laughter and no tears.

We are fortunate to be able to express our emotions, to show contentment and unhappiness. So what if today's laughter becomes tomorrow's tears? We know we'll laugh again — and cry again. Our past experiences give meaning to the present.

I will accept all my emotions as an affirmation of my life. Changing emotions are a part of normal living.

July 8

They do me wrong who say I come no more, / For every day I stand outside your door.

— Walter Malone

Opportunity doesn't just knock once, it's there all the time. Perhaps we just don't see it because we're frightened to try new things. Or we may be complacent. One of the ways we know we are really making capable, mature decisions is when we become willing to open the door to opportunity again.

Occasionally, when a person retires, he or she may expect life to become automatically wonderful — all the time in the world and nothing in particular to do. It may take a little time for us to adjust. Opportunity is always there, waiting. We can learn to open our own doors.

I can renew my energies by becoming eager to burst forward, to pursue leisure-time efforts, to work with others.

Should I, after tea and cakes and ices,
Have the strength to force the moment
to its crisis?
　　　　　— Thomas Stearns Eliot

Some people call it ''dancing around the issue.'' After all, if there is a problem to face, we may become embarrassed when it's time to talk about it. We try so hard to balance the emotional framework of our lives that we hardly want to be the one to bring up what seems to be a taboo topic. What we think, we don't always state; what we intend, we don't state clearly; and what we need, we rarely ask for. Our half-truths and mixed messages don't result in honest communication.

Drug use? Manipulative behavior? Eating disorder? Financial problems? The only way to begin to face a problem is to admit that there is one, to talk about it, and to decide together what steps can be taken to help.

Today, I will face a problem honestly.

July 10

It is costly wisdom that is bought by experience.

— *Roger Ascham*

Wisdom is gained in many ways. We can learn from others, if we're willing. We can listen to the voice within — that inner sense of what can and should be done. Or we can — and quite often do — pay the price for that wisdom gained from experience.

Sometimes, we ignore the cautioning voices of well-meaning friends and of our instincts, and leap instead onto foolhardy or dangerous ground. It might have to do with family problems or finances or even our personal care. Often if we fail, we pay a great price — in terms of relationships, money, or health. But even our failures are not wasted if from them we gain the wisdom of caution and care.

I will try to listen and learn from others and thereby save myself some pain.

The biggest thing in our today's sorrow is the memory of yesterday's joy.
— *Kahlil Gibran*

Even though we intellectually know that a chronic illness will never go away, we emotionally offer ourselves a small glimmer of hope of recovery, of our lives going on as before.

We may spend some time reviewing life's memories, closing out whole chapters, and dealing with how life used to be. Then we can open a whole new section of life that allows us to include pain and sickness as part of our days. We work in the frame of reference of today. This is today's problem, and we can work it into our lives. Acknowledging that we are living a part of our lives differently from before will be our first step toward adjustment. We accept, we change, and we begin to create new joys in the present to ease our sorrow.

By altering my goals, I once again can move into the mainstream of life.

July 12

There is a certain state of health that does not allow us to understand everything; and perhaps illness shuts us off from certain truths; but health shuts us off just as effectively from others.
— Andre Gide

When we were healthy, it was hard imagining what someone in poor health was going through. We could sympathize — even empathize — but we were insulated from the reality because we had no personal experience with illness.

Now, our diminished health allows us to put ourselves in someone else's shoes. Many of our friends and family don't always know how to act toward us or what to say. They're the ones who may be uneasy about facing our world. We can help them because we know what they are experiencing.

I will be compassionate to my loved ones as they strive to help and understand.

We often make self-defeating choices because we are unenlightened about our needs. We pick the opposite of what we really need because we don't know what we need.
— Lila Swell

Sometimes we may repeatedly engage in self-defeating behaviors. Poor work habits can lead to being fired and being defeated again. Overeating causes obesity, health issues, and poor image, which may lead to fad dieting and more failure. Until lightning strikes, until we finally realize that we are defeating our deepest needs — spiritual and emotional — we plod along on the same path.

The direction of our behavior changes when we see what our needs are and that they are the same for everyone. We all need love, compassion, and the opportunity to love others, and we can satisfy those needs in healthy ways.

I'll make positive choices for myself today.

July 14

Nothing is unthinkable, nothing impossible to the balanced person, provided it arises out of the needs of life and is dedicated to life's further developments.

— Lewis Mumford

Occasionally, we may be discouraged over the loss of an ability we'd always counted on. Accepting this loss often requires a major emotional adjustment.

Our lives need not be defined by our inabilities, but instead by our possibilities. If bogged down in negativity, we may truly become the *dis*-abled people that others see at first glance.

Marvelous opportunities for growth and joy often await us — through doors we can choose to open and pass through. Almost nothing is impossible if we want to get there badly enough.

I won't use medical problems as excuses to bow out of life. Today, I will look for opportunities for challenge and growth.

Let us then be up and doing, with a heart for any fate.
— *Henry Wadsworth Longfellow*

There may have been times in our lives when we have been forced, for one reason or another, to eat a bland diet. The reasons don't matter; what does matter is how totally bored we became with the unvarying beige-and-white soft menu! Before long we had lost our anticipation of eating.

We may sometimes place ourselves on a bland diet of life. Daily routine stays much the same, day after day, year after year. From home to work to the sofa to bed, and start all over again. Some routine is like a healthy diet that gives us stability and safety, but a sprinkling of risk is the seasoning that adds zest to our lives. We can reach out for what is not habit. We can continue to try when previous efforts have failed. We can take a generous helping of life.

I can dare to change or to try new things without sacrificing all of my routine and safety.

July 16

What is experience? A poor little hut constructed from the ruins of the palace of gold and marble called our illusion.

— *Joseph Roux*

Our youthful dreams of glory, adventure, and wealth have, for most of us, been unfulfilled, yet we are not disappointed. Childlike illusions that a meaningful life had to be based on excitement and power have given way to a maturity that values simpler, yet more important, goals.

Our long-ago need for importance was based on the judgment of others. We wanted other people to see our wealth, feel our power, possibly even envy our influence. Today, we seek our own approval. We value serenity, not adventure. Love, not envy. Acceptance, not power. We live with goals, not illusions.

I am thankful that my values are strong.

A thing of beauty is a joy forever:
Its loveliness increases; it will never
Pass into nothingness.
                                    — *John Keats*

We know a work of fine art can only increase in value. As the years pass by, art develops character lines which further define and highlight its beauty.

We wonder about people. There is grace which comes with age, we know, but how can people last forever? The answer, of course, is we do not. But all that we comprise and create — the love, the caring, the storytelling, the things we make with our hands — will endure forever. Just as enduring, and perhaps even more valuable, is the respect we give to our family and traditions. These and other family heirlooms are our assurance that no one or no thing passes into nothingness.

I am comforted by the traditions of family and faith and by the meaningfulness they add to my life.

July 18

Who controls the past controls the future; who controls the present controls the past.

— *George Orwell*

We planned on being healthy, on always being healthy, so our adjustment to less than optimal health can be quite difficult. Until we get our priorities back in gear, it can seem as though the scales are just not tipping in our favor.

Life can feel overwhelming when we foresee no apparent reprieve from our pain and inconvenience. It takes a while sometimes to learn to live with a health problem, but we can do it. With time we gain insight. Our lives are in our control once again.

We are responsible for ourselves, although sometimes we may forget that fact. Once we get a firm hold on our emotions, on our new set of problems, we understand that we still make the decisions for ourselves.

I can make positive decisions that alter the path of my life.

*Our faith comes in moments; our vice
is habitual.*
— *Ralph Waldo Emerson*

Some habits are not good for us, yet
we can fall into them so easily. "Just one
more drink," we rationalize. "It won't
hurt me. I don't have to go to work
tomorrow." "Just a small piece of cake.
I'll start my diet tomorrow." We may not
realize that we are acting in a pattern.
Being human, we continue in this way
until something happens which forces us
to change our patterns and ourselves.

Whatever that something is, it may
prompt many actions, one of which may
be to turn to our faith for solace. Many
things in our lives are uncertain. There is
uncertainty as to how our day will be. It
is our faith that keeps us going regardless
of any setbacks. The moments of darkness
we all fall into can be overcome by faith.

*I can believe and trust in my Higher Power no
matter what is happening in my life now.*

July 20

*We should not let our fears hold us
back from pursuing our hopes.*
— *John F. Kennedy*

Regardless of our situation, we all need
to hope. When we were young we were
in a hurry all the time. Every problem
needed a quick solution. And our anticipated futures were completely untarnished
by adult viewpoints.

Sometimes, what we mislabel as a fear
of dying might really be regret that we
haven't led a full enough life. We know
now what is reasonable and what is not.
We understand where we are in our lives
and accept that ideal situations may not
come to pass. We have learned that we
must come to terms with who we are and
what we can do. We have learned that we
are okay just as we are today.

*I have come to terms with where I am in my
life. My fears will not hold me back anymore.*

An hour of pain is as long as a day of pleasure.

— Proverb

When we look back at our lives, do the painful experiences come through first? We may remember the difficult times that led to the end of a relationship or losing a job. Life seemed at a standstill during those times, as we wondered whether we'd ever get close to another person, find another job, or feel confident again.

We probably learned much later that failures could be opportunities for growth. As we sift through our hardest memories, we can settle back into the happy ones again, knowing we have learned and grown from our pain. And as our ''hour'' of pain comes to an end, we can see the large and small pleasures of today and remember those of yesterday.

I will not let pain obscure my joys and pleasures.

July 22

*We must believe in the conquest of the
spirit of the world by the spirit of God.
But, the miracle must happen in us,
before it can happen in the world.*
— *Albert Schweitzer*

There is a time in the progression of life
or pain or illness when we realize that no
matter how extensive our resources are, no
matter how deep our emotional well, we
cannot depend only upon ourselves. We
all recognize that time when it's at hand;
no one has to inform us.

Even if our faith has been shaken before, we are able, once again, to reach
out to a Power greater than ourselves. Our
Higher Power offers reassurance that even
as we continue to adjust, even when we
have coped as well as we can, a greater
comfort and care is open to us.

*I can't control everything. I find freedom and
relief in knowing I don't have to.*

*A friend is clearer than the light of
heaven, for it would be better for us
that the sun were extinguished than
that we should be without friends.*
— *St. John Chrysostom*

Friendship is our greatest achievement
and reward. Our friends are people to care
about, celebrate with, and count on. Even
after the diagnosis of a chronic medical
condition, friends are there for each other.
Within the closest friendships we find the
best of each other at all times.

Friendships enrich our lives.   It is
no accident that we become close and
maintain our contact. Our paths crossed
for reasons, and we are forever a part
of each other's life.   We really listen.
We open up.   We offer help and hope.
We share each other's pain and enhance
each other's growth.   We appreciate our
friend's unique qualities.   We let each
other know who we really are.

I bring myself honestly to my friendships.

July 24

*Keep your fears to yourself but share
your courage with others.*
— *Robert Louis Stevenson*

Each of us harbors secret fears. "How
will I manage?" "Can I make it through
today?" "Will my family still love me if
my behavior has been inappropriate?"

We learn, rather early in the game, that
a defeatist attitude drives our friends away
after a period of time. Therefore, it's
often up to us to deal with our own fears.
We do our best to ease ourselves through
each crisis — and at times we will need
additional help — but by and large we can
do it. It isn't so much that we're overly
independent or angry. It's that we need
to help our loved ones learn how to cope
with our illness, so we keep our fears from
becoming irrational as best we can. And
that often passes for courage.

*I will put my fears into proper perspective be-
cause this helps me — and my loved ones.*

*He who knows others is learned, He
who knows himself is wise.*
                              — Lao Tsze

We sometimes let how we think we
should act keep us from showing our
deepest feelings. We may behave the way
others expect us to act, while burying
within ourselves the pain and fears associated with our changing health.

Acting upon our own thoughts and feelings can be difficult; acting according to
what others think is frustrating — and
impossible. Gradually we find more stability and confidence within ourselves. This
self-trust allows us to show our emotions
and to express our ideas and feelings. We
might be short-tempered sometimes, or
impatient, or angry. None of us is perfect. We accept that truth, and are freed of
the burden of pleasing others; we discover
the joy of acting on our inner messages of
growth and honesty.

*I am most free to grow when I am acting hon-
estly on my own values and feelings.*

July 26

The future is called "perhaps," which is the only possible thing to call the future. And the important thing is not to allow that to scare you.
— *Tennessee Williams*

"I'm going to work in the mills, like my Dad." "I'm going to be a teacher." "I want to be a soldier." As children, we believed in these absolute, fixed goals. In adulthood, we learn that we don't always get what we expect. Sometimes we don't even come close. Those who manage to live happy and fulfilling lives are flexible, mature adults.

Flexibility means we can incorporate changes into our lives, even when those changes cause a difference in the way we live. What's most important is to remember that we can change goals and attain them, that happiness is there if we work and plan for it.

I am not afraid to make changes that are good for me.

One of the signs of maturity is a healthy respect for reality — a respect that manifests itself in the level of one's aspirations and in the accuracy of one's assessment of the difficulties which separate the facts of today from the bright hopes of tomorrow.
— *Robert H. Davies*

If we don't want to live our lives caught in the ''what might have been'' doldrums, we can assess where we are and how we happen to be here. We can stop feeling regretful about lost time and concentrate on the possibilities now.

If we haven't achieved any of the goals we previously set for ourselves, we can make new goals and achieve each of them one step at a time. We have the rest of our lives to live, and we can realistically shape new goals that are both challenging and reachable.

I will set realistic goals, realizing there is never a better time than now.

July 28

Life is not a "brief candle." It is a splendid torch that I want to make burn as brightly as possible before handing it on to future generations.
— *George Bernard Shaw*

How lucky we are to have the splendid torch of our lives shining on our days. Some may think that a health problem is going to become a permanent barrier to our ability to enjoy life.

If we assume that each one of our "small candles" represents another of our strengths, we can blend them together to form a torch of hope. How we live the rest of our lives — forty months or forty years — is entirely our own making. Let the torch shine!

The possibilities of my life are endless when I am willing to see them and act on them.

Positive attitudes — optimism, high self-esteem, and outgoing nature, joy-ousness, and the ability to cope with stress — when established early in life, may be the most important basis for continued good health.
— Helen Hayes

Positive attitudes and high self-esteem are wonderful attributes, but not all of us are lucky enough to develop them early in our lives. Because we haven't developed strong coping strategies doesn't mean we don't have the opportunity now. It's hard to change, and we can only do it if it becomes important for us to make the effort.

When we are going through stressful times, especially those times related to a health problem, we can develop our courage by acting ''as if'' we have high self-esteem, ''as if'' we can cope well. Remarkably, we may find that we do.

A time of high stress has forced me to face my own character deficits. I am working on developing positive attitudes.

July 30

There is nothing which we receive
with so much reluctance as advice.
                    — Joseph Addison

As children, most of us were unrecep-
tive to advice. Our parents offered words
of warning and frequently we refused to
hear because we needed independence.

Today, when friends or family members
make suggestions, we might have some of
the same reactions as we did as children.
We still need independence, and some
advice — no matter how well meant —
carries with it the implication that we are
less than capable of clearly seeing dangers
or knowing our options. We're better able
now to weigh the messages we receive. We
have two choices. When our loved ones
offer suggestions that we know to be bad
or inappropriate for us, we can remind
ourselves that they are meant well and
merely say thank you. When the advice
is good, we can do the same thing.

I will listen carefully to all the loving advice given
me.

*From happiness to suffering is a step;
from suffering to happiness is an
eternity.*

— *Jewish Proverb*

The loss of normal good health can rock
even the strongest person. In one frag-
ile moment our life seems in shambles.
All that we anticipated, all that we had
planned, seems over forever. We wonder
if we'll ever get through this suffering.

For a while it may seem as though we
are living underwater — nothing is clear
or straightforward. The things that once
gave us pleasure seem to disappear as grief
takes their place. Friends offer to help
— and they do help for a time — but
ultimately we face our loss alone.

Finally we begin to understand that
grief is a process, just as life is a process.
We will be able to move toward acceptance and serenity, and eventually we can
be happy again. We can continue to live.

*I am consoled in knowing grief takes time, but
it will end. I can continue to grow.*

August

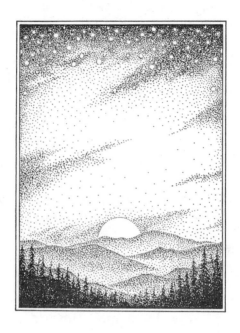

Oft when the white still dawn
Lifted the skies
and pushed the hills apart
I have felt it like glory in my heart.
    — *Edwin Markham*

The world is one, a whole, and we are a part of it. But sometimes, we are so enmeshed in ourselves — in the details of our lives, in the unfair limitations placed upon us — that we become closed and forget the rest of the world. We see nothing else. We hear nothing else.

But if we reenter the world, the natural balance there gives us peace and comfort. The beauty — splashes of color, fragrance of flowers, trees swaying in a breeze — is also our beauty. We inhale the breath of spring amid the sounds of life. All seems right with the world, and we are one with all life.

Today, I will find joy and meaning in being alive within a living world.

August 2

*No man is good for anything who has
not some particle of obstinacy to use
upon occasion.*
— *Henry Ward Beecher*

The word *obstinate* is quite often used to
describe children who refuse to let go of
an idea or behavior. Although we may not
want others to label us obstinate, it might
be that obstinacy is a needed quality for
us in the right situations.

Sometimes it is healthy for us to be
stubborn, to hold steadfastly to what we
want and who we are and where we want
to be. Faith in ourselves and obstinacy can
be just what we need to survive a hard
day. And we do get by, not because we're
foolish, but because our maturity tells us
to hold on to our sense of direction.

I will keep as much independence as I can.

Somewhere along the line of development we discover what we really are, and then we make our real decision for which we are responsible.
— *Eleanor Roosevelt*

Many of us have begun to reexamine our lives and our values. Am I proud of how I act? Of what I do? Will this decision be in my best interest? Do I have strong, interacting relationships?

A likely result of this might be that we fool ourselves less now and that we don't try to fool others. The discovery of what we really are and of what is important to us urges us toward greater honesty. We are freer to make amends to friends and family members for things we've said or done. We hesitate less in asking for help and in telling others when we feel wronged. Best of all, we've rid ourselves of our old victim mentality and have taken responsibility for our lives.

I will begin happily to make responsible decisions today.

August 4

Today is the day in which to express your noblest qualities of mind and heart, to do at least one worthy thing which you have long postponed. . . .
— *Grenville Kleiser*

Volunteer work. There are volunteer jobs for people with every level of ability. The main qualification is to care about others. Each day offers us the opportunity to make a difference in someone else's life. We may choose to sing in a community choir or play in an amateur band. Or we might offer to read stories to or write letters for people with limited vision.

Volunteer work. What's remarkable are the benefits we will reap from the simple act of sharing our abilities, our lives, our caring. These acts affirm the bond that exists between us. They help us move out of a preoccupation with ourselves and our limitations, and they put us into the mainstream of life.

Today, I will share my abilities and talents with others.

*My handicap is part of me because I
have had to make peace with it. And
in doing so, I've made peace with the
less obvious handicaps of other people,
like resentment, prejudice, hate.*
— *Ginger Hutton*

Living with an illness — whether our
own or a loved one's — has taught us that
handicaps are not always physical. We
begin to understand fear is handicapping,
prejudice is handicapping, inaccessibility
to the community is handicapping.

More and more we are able to make
peace with our own limitations and those
of others, and as we do this we gain insight into which of them we have to accept
and which we don't. We recognize there
are some limitations we can do something
about and others we must accept for the
sake of our serenity.

*The more tolerant I am, the less limited I
become.*

August 6

> *Believe, when you are most unhappy,*
> *that there is something for you to do in*
> *the world. So long as you can sweeten*
> *another's pain, life is not in vain.*
> — Helen Keller

Day-to-day problems can become so overwhelming that we just can't fathom how we will manage. At those times, the three most difficult things to do might be the very things we should do.

First, we must admit to ourselves that we are, indeed, in an emotional crisis. Then, we should reach out to the community for support. People never know we need help if we don't ask. A nearly endless array of services is in place for us — grief groups, counseling, AA, Al-Anon, Overeaters Anonymous, and other Twelve Step groups. Thirdly, we have the option of moving beyond ourselves and reaching out to someone else who suffers.

It's within my power to help myself by connecting with people who care.

Eat little at night, open your windows, drive out often, and look for the good in things and people. . . . You will no longer be sad, or bored, or ill.
— Mary Knowles

When we get caught up in our problems, it may seem that they will continue to escalate, repeat, and escalate again. We all have hard times — times when we are uncertain whether or not life has meaning, and at those times it may feel as though we have no control over the direction or quality of our lives.

But when we ease back a little and remember the hundreds of small choices we can make, we're more able to accept some of the large, unchangeable realities of our lives. We can't cure ourselves or change other people, but we can make the choices and take charge of the decisions that are ours.

I can simplify my life by letting go of decisions and problems that aren't mine to handle.

August 8

Man can do much for himself as respects his own improvement, unless self-love so blinds him that he cannot see his own imperfections and weaknesses.

— Martha Wilson

Remember Hide and Seek? Oleeey oleeey in free? What wonderful times they were when we were so certain we could hide from others. Now we are adults, and one would think we are no longer hiding. That's not, unfortunately, always true. Many of us hide within negative behaviors which become habits.

Looking at our own weaknesses is a difficult task. We understand we have character defects, but we're afraid to change our familiar patterns. If we can admit there is a problem, we've taken the first step. Wanting to change comes next. Finally, we won't be hiding anymore.

Self-improvement is within my reach if I admit my negative behavior.

*Usually when people are sad, they
don't do anything. They just cry over
their condition. But when they get
angry, they bring about a change.*
— *Malcolm X*

Those of us who have a chronic illness
often feel a lot of anger, but we can choose
how to deal with the anger. If we insist on
denying it, we may isolate ourselves and
be numbed by an unbearable sadness. Or
we might lash out at the people we love.

A sounder choice for us is to acknowledge our anger — and our right to be angry. We don't deserve illness. Or pain.
When we allow ourselves these honest reactions, we are freer to move toward acceptance — and action. When we accept
our limitations — no matter how unfair
they are — we then can decide where
and how and when we will make needed
changes in our lives.

*My anger can lead me toward growth if I use it
in the right ways.*

August 10

Few men are so miserable as not to
like to talk of their misfortunes. . . .
— *Maria Edgeworth*

"Don't get stuck in a conversation with
Harry. He'll bore you to death telling
you his problems." We have all had the
experience of being warned away from a
certain person. There have probably even
been times when we were the "Harry"
others tried to avoid. It's normal to dwell
on our troubles, and we all like to talk
about them. There is an added responsibility on our shoulders now that there is a
medical problem present.

We can minimize that problem by becoming aware of what we are doing and
by saving our long medical conversations
for the people who really care and need
to know. Otherwise, we will find that our
friends will slip away, uncertain of how to
bear the burden of our changed health.

Caution will become my watchword as I learn to
live with my altered health patterns.

*Before an important decision someone
clutches your hand — a glimpse of
gold in the iron-gray, the proof of all
you have never dared to believe.*
— *Dag Hammarskjold*

There is nothing quite as lonely as having to make a decision. Imagine the feelings a family goes through when a beloved pet has to be put to sleep. The parents, because they truly understand the situation, must be the decision makers. If we are considering a job change, it will affect our immediate family and our friendships.

When a person extends a helping hand, we welcome it as a starving person would welcome food, for it offers affirmation and empathy. The decision is still difficult, but we have the inner strength to carry us through.

I believe in myself, but will welcome the support of others in my decision making.

August 12

Life is so full of miseries, minor and major. . . .
— *Agnes Repplier*

Occasionally a person who has chronic pain spends far too much time on a quest to cure or solve the pain. Support groups become much more than an extension of helpful purpose; they can become our total purpose. All the day can be filled with seeking the "right" people to solve our problems. All semblance of a well-balanced life gets pushed away.

There's no reason to make our days miserable with unrealistic goals. Learning to live the best we can with the pain and inconvenience of illness is the only way to make minor miseries out of major ones.

I can keep myself emotionally whole by seeking balance in my life.

*If you allow men to use you for your
own purposes, they will use you for
theirs.*

— *Aesop*

When we attend a party, isn't it always
the person with the cast or someone who
just had surgery who gets all the attention?
At first, when our health changes, we may
try to play other people for sympathy.

We finally begin to understand that
most of us have different needs. Ours
are more permanent than the needs of a
person with a broken leg. Upon realizing this, we could become angry that our
needs aren't being anticipated. After being ill for a while, we realize it's up to us
to let others know what we are feeling and
what our needs are. Then we can look for
understanding, not pity.

*Exploiting the role of "sick person" is one be-
havior I need to guard against. I will accept this
as a personal challenge.*

August 14

Physical strength can never permanently withstand the impact of spiritual force.
— *Franklin D. Roosevelt*

It's a peculiar twist of life that physical impairment causes some of us to become either agnostic or more spiritual. Few of us stay in the shades of gray.

Those of us who are fortunate enough to find our Higher Power or to rediscover our sense of spirituality may feel a deep and abiding belief in spiritual forces which will dwell with us at all times in our lives.

Spirituality transcends all health problems; we can call on its comfort and support at will. Our beliefs can buoy us up when we are feeling low and can richly enhance all the facets of our lives.

The spiritual forces which work within me are uniquely mine — to share or to keep private. They will always enhance my life.

*As we advance in life, we learn the
limits of our abilities.*

— J. A. Froud

Remember the lofty goals we had when
we were young? Goals that included being
the best, saving all the children, having a
lot of money. We could be president, put
out fires, or be on stage. We could accomplish anything when we were young.
The older we got, the more realistic we
became. We began to be aware of what
we couldn't do, of the fact that not every family system worked, that not every
person was happy.

We found new goals then, goals that we
could live with for that time in our lives.
Even now, as we read, we are learning
about ourselves. We know that we may
not reach our childhood goals. We have
learned our limits and are living our lives
in a realistic fashion.

*Awareness of my own limits has helped me set
realistic goals. I am successful.*

August 16

Be not afraid of life. Believe that life is worth living and your belief will help create the fact.
— *William James*

The words ''life is worth living'' may seem inappropriate to someone who has a serious personal conflict. A pat on the shoulder or a hug just isn't enough to convince us that all we are going through makes life ''worth living.''

A sense of worthiness is an ongoing process. And the value of life is affirmed and strengthened by our willingness to listen to our emotional and physical needs — especially when we feel unhappy or unhealthy. That willingness is shown in action. A cup of coffee and a good cry with a close friend, acceptance of our Higher Power's wisdom and care, or seeking help from a trained professional — all of these actions say, ''I and my life have worth.''

By helping myself, I will act on my belief that life is worth living.

*Sadness is almost never anything but
a form of fatigue.*
— *Andre Gide*

There are times in every life when the road gets a little bumpy. Occasionally we become so overwhelmed with work, with life in general, that we become exhausted. With the fatigue can come sadness — sadness at not being able to work the way we expected to, sadness at not looking or feeling as well as we want to, or sadness caused by grieving. We may feel sorry for ourselves or feel nearly paralyzed by fatigue.

We can recognize that fatigue is one of the many forms that sadness takes. Feelings of sorrow or helplessness can be diminished by confiding them to a friend or to a physician. We can only be as well as we expect to be — as well as we allow ourselves to be.

When I feel very fatigued or sad, I can be open and honest about my problem. Hiding behind fatigue only causes sadness.

August 18

*You may judge others only according
to your knowledge of yourself.*
                    — *Kahlil Gibran*

We know that our behavior patterns may not be the only acceptable ones. Many of us have spent the major part of our lives trying to please others. Now we are learning to please ourselves. We finally understand that there's no need for us to reach beyond our own capabilities.

Now that our physical health is limited and our emotional health is stretched almost to the breaking point, we begin to realize that people around us may have serious problems of their own. By reaching out, unselfishly, we can help. Inadvertently, we will reap the benefits of our own behavior.

As I understand my limitations, I begin to know myself more intimately than ever before. I am learning about my untapped potential.

*The past should be culled like a box
of fresh strawberries, rinsed of debris,
sweetened judiciously and served in
small portions, not very often.*
— *Laura Palmer*

Many of us may dwell in the past,
telling ourselves our yesterdays were better than our tomorrows will ever be. Living in "what was" can be dangerous, for
we may be less adaptable to life's changes.

Fond memories are healthy when they
remind us how our lives are formed and
shaped by our experiences. Memories re-
veal our development into the productive
people we are today. Life does get better
every day because we have both the joys
of the present and some sweet memories
of the past. We not only survive, we regain happiness and our peace of mind by
living for today and by appreciating all the
todays and yesterdays.

*I will not live in the past, but instead will look
to each day as new and promising.*

*Repose is not more welcome to the
worn and to the aged, to the sick
and to the unhappy, than danger,
difficulty, and toil, to the young and
the adventurous.*

— *Fanny Burney*

Within the same week, a ten-year-old
boy made a solo flight across America,
and a woman who was over eighty climbed
Mount Everest. Some of us don't aspire to
such mind-boggling events. But there is a
time for more adventurous quests and a
time for quiet. They don't have to be age-
related.

Sometimes our concern about age may
be more limiting than our physical capabilities. "Should a person my age be
acting like this?" "I think I'm too old
for that." Thoughts like these prevent us
from exploring and learning and acquiring
new skills. We can choose our direction,
regardless of age.

*I will set aside age prejudice when I look at the
possibilities before me today.*

Nothing can bring you peace but yourself.
— *Ralph Waldo Emerson*

True peace comes from the harmony we feel within ourselves. We don't go out and get peace of mind; it's the result of what we do. Harmony is being at ease with ourselves, our surroundings, and with our lives. This is no easy task, as we must come to grips with the issues that cause us concern.

This doesn't mean that all our problems must be solved before we can have inner peace, for life will be much like a mountain road, with twists and turns and many unexpected bumps. Peace is a reality for those who accept what cannot be changed and take up the challenges that can and must be dealt with. Peace is easier to attain when we cherish the gifts of the present moment.

In my life, peace begins with me. I will remember that peace is a prize of the spirit and is available to everyone.

August 22

I have gout, asthma, and seven other
maladies, but am otherwise very well.
— *Sydney Smith*

We may be awed by people who are able
to handle any problem that comes their
way. They seem to have a magic touch.
They are strong, we think, and they seem
to so easily separate their emotional and
spiritual selves from what happens to them
physically.

There are people who can always manage to find happiness. Indeed, they often
can find laughter in the midst of chaos.
We may feel jealous of their apparent ability to handle troubles. Often, however, we
learn that they have come through terri-
ble life crises, abusive relationships, bouts
with cancer, or chronic health difficulties.
The ones we envy may have learned, the
hard way, that each problem must be handled on its merit. There is no magic touch,
just touching experiences.

I may have problems, but I can allow myself the
right to be otherwise well.

So never let a cloudy day ruin your sunshine, for even if you can't see it, the sunshine is still there, inside of you, ready to shine when you will let it.

— Amy Michelle Pitzele

Amazing words of wisdom sometimes spring from the mouths of children. This child was just nine years old when she wrote these words, which are the last stanza of a poem about understanding change. Life seen through the eyes of a child can be serenely simplistic. Where does a child get that kind of wisdom and that depth of understanding?

We can struggle to keep the child in us alive. We, too, can recognize that even when the cloudy days come, the sunshine — our smiles, our hopes, our dreams — is still there, ready to beam at a moment's notice.

Today, my own personal sun will shine within me, no matter what the weather is outside.

August 24

Faults are thick where love is thin.
— *James Howell*

We often overlook the faults of people we love. Sometimes, in fact, our love so blinds us that we don't have to overlook their faults, because we don't even see them. Yet if our love wavers or if a friendship begins to weaken, it may seem as though our friends have developed numerous flaws or maddening habits.

When this happens, we learn to reassess our relationship and ourselves. Rather than conclude that our loved one has become less than he or she was before, we know that change has occurred within us. Then we decide whether the friendship is important enough to try to rebuild it. Sometimes it is, and we work to recapture the trust and communication we once had. Sometimes it isn't, and we decide to let go of it and, in doing so, let go of resentment and fault-finding.

The decision to rebuild or to let go of friendships often rests with me.

Sometimes it is more important to discover what one cannot do, than what one can do.

— Lin Yutang

Understanding limitations is important in our lives. As we mature, we naturally let go of old dreams and develop new ones. We start to reexamine, to set priorities, to find out what we are capable of, and what we are still able to accomplish. Finally, we understand that we may not be the tallest, the richest, the handsomest, or the most intelligent.

We learn how to find what is normal for us, how to establish a new balance in our lives. We learn to accept who we are. Acceptance of change in our lives includes those changes that occur with chronic health problems. This is one of our most difficult challenges, but we will grow in our ability to cope with this illness too.

I continually struggle to find the new balance in my life, but I know it's a growth process of which I'm capable.

August 26

Friendship: A ship big enough to carry two in fair weather, but only one in foul.

— *Ambrose Bierce*

Let's be honest. When we have a choice, don't we avoid aggravation, fear, and pain in our friendships? Before we judge friends and family members who have been unable to cope with our chronic condition, we should ask ourselves to understand their choice. Certainly, we wouldn't choose to have the pain, inconvenience, and limitations of our illnesses if we had the same choice as they do.

Most of us have been hurt by friends who have abandoned us because of our medical conditions, but it might be time now for us to forgive them. We can remind ourselves that abandonment does not mean our friends were unloving or uncaring; it only means they selected an option that we don't have.

I will work to forgive those who have left me.

*The essence of optimism is that it ...
enables a man to hold his head high,
to claim the future for himself and not
abandon it to his enemy.*
— *Dietrich Bonhoeffer*

"She always looks to the sour side,"
we've heard it said, or "He always has a
pleasant smile." The difference, as we all
know, between an optimist and a pessimist
is entirely in their attitudes. A pessimist
sees little, if anything, to look forward to
in life. In that case, life is tediously lived.
If we think in positive ways, we see the
good. That good becomes the primary part
of our lives.

An optimist, regardless of personal
problems, is eager to arise in the morning — to get to work, to be with friends
or family, to live the happiness of the day.
People are drawn toward optimists, for
their joy shines on everyone around them.

*Life is an adventure of choices to be lived, not
an ordeal to be survived. I choose optimism and
joy.*

August 28

Pain is life — the sharper, the more evidence of life.
— Charles Lamb

We all have pain in our lives. This is not necessarily illness, but deeper emotional pain caused by our perception of failure or success. Caused by a relationship ending. Caused by loss. Caused by giving up unrealistic goals. We all experience pain.

We gain the knowledge that pain broadens our base of experience and can make us stronger — or weaker. And we are the ones who ultimately have to carry the burden and joy of our lives.

There's more here than "pain in life." It's how we learn to handle our pain, how we react to what has caused our pain, and how we have made others feel about our pain that matters the most.

I choose to be a survivor. My experiences can enrich my life.

*Lord, teach us to number our days,
that we may apply our hearts unto
wisdom.*

— *Psalm 90*

Funny, but when we were kids we probably didn't give much thought to words
such as *peace* or *harmony*. We just lived
our sweet childish lives with little, if any,
worry about feelings.

Now we speak often of ''meeting of the
minds,'' ''harmonious thoughts,'' and
''world peace,'' for we all want to achieve
as high a level of personal and emotional comfort as we are able. With our
newly developed understanding of wisdom
comes a deepened sense of pride because
we know that each day is a precious entity,
special in and of itself.

*The harmony and peace that surround me are
mine for the taking.*

August 30

> *The basic fact of today is the tremendous pace of change in human life.*
> — *Jawaharlal Nehru*

Just when we convince ourselves that we are settled, something happens that causes us to change once again. We need to become chameleons, open to change and willing to adapt.

It's not a simple process, for sometimes life throws us zingers we never expected. Not all change is positive, and it can be downright hard. Perhaps we may become grandparents quite unexpectedly, or we may need to move to a different city. We can lose a spouse or a job or our health. All these situations cause further change. Rising to the occasion teaches us that we are, finally, truly adult in our behavior.

I let go of old dreams each time I change. I am proud of my ability to adapt to new circumstances.

A mature person is one who does not think only in absolutes, who is able to be objective even when deeply stirred emotionally. . . .
— *Eleanor Roosevelt*

Many of us are well aware of how easily tempers flare or tears can flow when we face an unexpected problem or situation. Perhaps illness contributes to this sensitivity, but we might also consider whether we've become more rigid. Are we holding too tightly to absolutes, wanting to have the right answer or the right response to almost everything? Has coping with unpredictable illnesses driven us to seek predictability in other areas of our lives?

Maturity often means letting go of the need to control. We also find greater peace by allowing ourselves to be unprepared for people and events we can't prepare for. There are no absolutes, and we don't have to live as though there were.

I will be willing to consider new ideas.

September

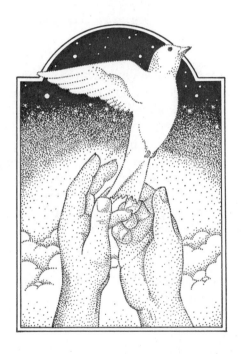

*Spirituality is like a bird: if you hold
on to it tightly, it chokes, and if you
hold it loosely, it escapes.*
— *Israel Salanter Lipkin*

Being spiritual does not necessarily
mean being religious. Instead, it can be an
awakening of our deepest personal sense
of caring about other people, as well as an
awakening of our appreciation of the joy,
symmetry, and balance of nature.

The spirituality we strive for and which
comforts us best is based on our finding
a similar balance within ourselves. When
we possessively clutch our faith and expect all that we demand, our spirituality
is weakened. Yet, if we expect nothing of
it, it might seem to disappear. Our spiritual lives are strengthened as we find that
precious balance between expectant trust
in our Higher Power and responsible re-
liance on ourselves.

*I am striving to find fullness and balance in my
days. Certain experiences change the balance,
but I can find it again.*

September 2

My coat and I live comfortably together. It has assumed all my wrinkles, does not hurt me anywhere, has molded itself on my deformities, and is complacent to all my movements. I only feel its presence because it keeps me warm.

— *Victor Hugo*

The anticipation of school beginning each fall is fueled by youngsters' love of newness — new clothes, new shoes, new books, new teachers. We still enjoy newness, but we also find comfort in what is old and reliable. No afghan comforts quite as well as the one that was knitted with loving hands many years ago. We may have a favorite mug or chair. Over the years we have developed trusting and dependable relationships. While we remain open to change, we also feel comfortable with what is old and familiar.

I'm glad I can find comfort in the old and familiar, and excitement in the new and unfamiliar.

My message is peace of mind, not curing cancer, blindness, or paraplegia. . . . Anyone who is willing to work at it can achieve it.
— *Bernie S. Siegel*

Too often, we think we can regain our peace of mind only after our health problems are resolved. But peace of mind is what we need right now, not later. We can do a few things in our medical treatment, but we can actively develop our spiritual and emotional strengths.

We can look at life not in terms of success or failure, but in terms of attitudes and beliefs and self-acceptance. We can reprioritize our life goals to emphasize what can be done. Gradually, we experience a sense of peace as we separate those things which we can change and control from those which we can not. Making our choices and acting upon them brings us the peace we need in difficult times.

I will consider only the choices that are truly mine to make.

September 4

> *I learned that nothing is impossible*
> *when we follow our inner guidance,*
> *even when its direction may threaten*
> *us by reversing our usual logic.*
> — Gerald G. Jampolsky

Two voices play about our heads. We hear, ''Do it the way you've always done it,'' and the opposing, ''Take a chance — you can do it a different way.'' Sometimes we have to take a chance — on ourselves, on finding a better way.

What if we walk a new, longer, less convenient path home? What if we abandon the unsuccessful patterns we've followed with our loved ones? What if we speak our minds, rather than remain silent? Good things can happen when we dare to change. And if nothing happens? We would still have the pleasure of a new way home, of communicating on a different level, of knowing the joy of daring to change.

When I follow my inner voice my opportunities are endless.

*No faith is our own that we have not
arduously won.*
— *Havelock Ellis*

Everything that touches our lives influences our level of trust and spirituality. There are times when our faith, especially in ourselves, goes astray. This may be caused by losing a job, losing our good health, a negative change in a relationship. Our faith can be shaken when the things we expected to always be there are suddenly gone.

We can begin to regain that faith by remembering our Higher Power is constant, even when our faith is not. We humans fluctuate between doubt and trust, but that doesn't diminish the care that is always available to us. We need only surrender to that truth, and we find comfort.

My faith — in myself and in my Higher Power — is built upon my awareness that I don't have to struggle alone. I am strengthened when I admit to my spiritual needs.

September 6

Lie down and listen to the crabgrass grow, the faucet leak, and learn to leave them so.

— Marya Mannes

Sometimes we are driven by a need to get everything done. We have an inner sense of what we should be, and we work toward meeting that expectation. But we may strive beyond those goals because of what we believe our friends, our co-workers, and even the advertising media expect of us.

Only we can decide which expectations to satisfy. But first, we must be sure that the things we strive for are really our needs and goals. If an alphabetized spice rack or an organized workbench gives us no satisfaction, why should we alphabetize or organize? If an imperfect lawn doesn't bother us, we can let go of our concern and let the crabgrass grow.

Today, I will hold on only to my goals and expectations. I will let go of those which give me no joy.

No great thing is created suddenly.
— *Epictetus*

It took many thousands of years for the Seven Wonders of the World to form, and they are truly awe-inspiring. We, too, can create great things, but we must be patient as the results of our efforts slowly evolve.

We can participate in the creation of a strong family as one of our great wonders, for a loving, close, caring family extends beyond the present generation. The love and family traditions we help create will be handed down from generation to generation. It's not so important that we see at once the greatness of what we do. What does matter is that we are able to make an effort and know that the reward will take time.

I can patiently work toward the creation of new ideas and traditions, knowing that rewards will be apparent in time.

September 8

Every great mistake has a halfway moment, a split second when it can be recalled and perhaps remedied.
— *Pearl S. Buck*

We've all made decisions we've regretted. Regret doesn't change things, but we can learn to make better decisions in the future. Often there are moments in our decision-making process — especially in relationships — when we can still change our minds. At those times, we can reconsider what we want to say or do. Is it important enough to jeopardize a friendship? Sometimes it is, and that can't be helped.

But usually we discover we do want to preserve the relationship. We owe it to ourselves and our friends to look again, to think again, about what is being discussed or argued or decided. Sometimes, winning or being right isn't as important as the relationship.

I will take time to decide what is important and what isn't.

*God grant me the serenity to accept
the things I cannot change, courage
to change the things I can, and the
wisdom to know the difference.*
— *The Serenity Prayer*

The Serenity Prayer has comforted millions of people who strive to cope with change, disappointments, chemical dependency, and all sorts of other problems. This prayer can comfort us as we deal with the realities of chronic illness.

When we're overcome with pain or disappointed about slow or little progress, this prayer can help us put our lives into focus. It helps us see if we're wasting time and energy on things we can't change, such as the chronic conditions we live with, how others feel, and the past. And just as important, this prayer points us toward the things that we can control — our attitude, our willingness to change, and the outcome of this day.

*I pray for the wisdom to recognize the difference
between things I can and cannot change.*

September 10

The real world is not easy to live in.
It is rough; it is slippery.
                    — *Clarence Day*

What if the doctor has warned that the extra one hundred pounds is really going to cause death — imminently? What if the teenager who has been threatening to commit suicide succeeds? Does it take a crisis to shock us into action?

Too often we wait for an emergency situation to change our patterns of behavior. We can't change everything, but we do have it in our power to take back that which is in our control — our behavior.

We can take responsibility for our health, for our personal growth, and for our spiritual lives. We do not need to wait for an emergency.

Rather than waiting for a crisis to spur me into change, I can take positive action on my own.

*The world improves people according
to the dispositions they bring into it.*
— *Renier Giustina Michiel*

Remember the phrase, "Suck a sour lemon"? We have all known people who always look as though the world has handed them a bushel of lemons. No matter what the situation, no matter how happy other people would feel, these sour folks always have a reason to grimace.

Then there are the opposite kind — the ones who are dripping with sugar all the time. It doesn't matter how difficult their situation is, they always find reasons to smile. Both types are highly irritating and unrealistic, for life isn't always sweet and it's not always sour.

We can combine the two personality traits into a caring, compassionate human being who understands the highs and lows of life and who acts appropriately.

I can enhance my personal feelings of well-being by improving how I act toward others.

September 12

There is no more certain sign of a narrow mind, of stupidity, and of arrogance, than to stand aloof from those who think differently from us.
— *Walter Savage Landor*

We all carry some opinions and beliefs formed long ago, with no thought as to how they continue to affect us. We may be inflexible to beliefs or ideas that differ from ours. Because of this we might be intolerant of other people, especially those who seem different from us.

Our beliefs and actions toward other people may come from fear — a fear of the unexpected, of the unknown, or of being wrong. We may resist examining the rules and beliefs governing our lives because we're not totally sure of them. Opening ourselves to new ideas is easier if we remind ourselves that we don't have to accept the ideas, just the people.

I can fearlessly open myself to new ideas and new people.

*What next? Why ask? Next will come
a demand about which you already
know all you need to know: that its
sole measure is your own strength.*
— *Dag Hammarskjold*

Life is full of demands; we know and
expect that. Most of us wish we knew
about them ahead of time, but it's just
not possible to prepare in advance for
stress. Negative stressors like a flat tire or
a severe illness and positive stressors like a
family reunion are typical of the demands
placed on us throughout our lives.

Somehow, when these things happen,
we manage to rise to the occasion. We
may need to use all our resources — physical and spiritual — to cope, but we usually find within ourselves the strength and
enthusiasm for the demands we face.

*By knowing that I will be able to handle life's
crises with deep inner strength, I need not ask
myself "What's next?" anymore.*

September 14

I loafe and invite my soul,
I lean and loafe at my ease
observing a spear of summer grass.
                    — *Walt Whitman*

Sometimes we may have wished we could be like Aladdin and have three wishes. We might have even made mental lists of the things we could ask for.

We know that just having material possessions is not a guarantee for happiness. We know there has to be a purpose to life beyond wealth, a reason to get out of bed each morning. Whatever our walk of life, whatever our state of health, we all need to feel worthwhile.

We can't rub magic lanterns, but we can create important reasons for living, such as a paid job, volunteer work, gardening or another hobby, or just plain relaxing. Idleness is sometimes good for improving our attitude.

The power of relaxation is a strong reason to keep me from becoming stressed.

*A fanatic is one who can't change his
mind and won't change the subject.*
— *Winston Churchill*

Nearly everyone who has ever undergone a time of high stress has an intense need to talk about it. A person who has lost someone close may talk almost constantly about it. People who are admitting that they must deal with chronic pain often feel the same need.

We can and should expect our friends to allow us the comfort of talking about our feelings and experiences. As people who are suffering from pain and who are often driven to recount an illness' history, we need to realize there is a point at which people no longer want to listen — they may want to leave instead. We must work — harder than we ever have before — to build a well-balanced life that has some happy or humorous stories to share.

I will leave room in my conversations for stories that make me and my friends feel good.

September 16

Made weak by time and fate, but strong in will to strive, to seek, to find and not to yield.
— *Alfred, Lord Tennyson*

Some privacy is given up when we develop a chronic illness, for doctors and nurses need to know details of our medical histories. We can develop new strengths to offset this loss — pride that we are taking care of ourselves, and knowledge about our medical condition.

Many of the private battles we fight concern our feelings about having a chronic health problem. We may have to yield on some points — privacy, dependence, time, and energy — but we can continue to make personal gains in spite of our health.

Just because my health has changed does not mean I need to yield on points which matter to my well-being.

Fight one more round. When your feet are so tired you have to shuffle back to the center of the ring, fight one more round.

— *James J. Corbett*

One of the problems we most frequently hear about when a person is ill, whether it be mentally or physically, is exhaustion. We tell our doctors, our friends, anyone who will lend a willing ear, ''I'm just so very tired.''

To live in the fullest sense of the word, we have to, first of all, take care of ourselves. If what we feel is physical exhaustion, then we must allow ourselves the needed rest. We don't have to take on additional projects or commitments to prove ourselves. If, however, our tiredness has an emotional base, we may have to push ourselves — for just one more hour, for just one more day — trusting that the energy will come.

I will take care of myself this day. I am getting stronger, emotionally and spiritually.

September 18

*Our souls are hungry for meaning,
for the sense that we have figured out
how to live so that our lives matter,
so that the world [will] be at least
a little bit different for our having
passed through.*
— Harold Kushner

Even when we are no longer well, many of us continue to hunger for learning. We reach out to connect with other people and with book learning.

We continue to search on a deeper level as well. Not surprisingly, spirituality often takes a back seat, for a while, to the rigors of getting used to a changed medical condition. Ultimately, our souls cry out for growth just as our minds do, and we turn to our Higher Power for comfort and understanding.

My diminished health does not affect my drive for meaning and for learning. I want and need to learn.

Of a truth, men are mystically united:
a mystic bond of brotherhood makes
all men one.

— *Thomas Carlyle*

At our parent's knee we listened, enraptured, as we heard tales of how life used to be. We could hardly believe that they had lived sooooo long. As we moved into our teens, perhaps our parents became pathetically inept in our eyes, not to regain their intelligence until we were older.

Now we see that our folks were able to learn from their mistakes and move forward — just as we move forward now. We have learned ''what goes around comes around,'' and history repeats itself. Our parents imparted their greatest knowledge to us, and lovingly shared with us their mistakes so we could benefit.

I will listen with respect to the ones I love. I learn from them.

September 20

The natural wish of every human be-
ing, the weakest as well as the wisest,
seems to be, to leave some memorial
of themselves to posterity.
— *Susan Edmonstone Ferrier*

Each of us wants to leave evidence of our having lived. To perpetuate our names, we may work and play hard all our lives, or we may attempt to fine-tune sports skills or handcrafts.

We become gradually aware that material records of our lives will merely note our names and dates; they will not record who we are and what we value. The essence of each of us is found in each day, each moment. It is in living each day fully that we proclaim our worth and reflect it to our loved ones. What really matters, we realize, is how we spend our present, not how we try to manipulate the future. Living richly today is our memorial.

I will use today as a complete gift unto itself, not as a small brick for a future monument.

*. . . Summer coming to an end. So
we all try to keep it awake and stretch
it out by squeezing in all the boating,
picnicking, swimming. Sun, I crave
all year.*

— *Sister Mary Kraemer*

As the days begin to shorten and become cooler, we may suddenly be struck by the realization that the summer is over. With that thought might come the need to fill the last warm days with the many activities we postponed or, perhaps, forgot. At times like these, we may sense the need to hang on a little longer to the summer.

We do the same thing in other areas of our lives. At the moment we realize we are about to lose something very precious, that is when we value it most. Just before a dear friend moves away, we try to fill our days with togetherness. Knowing this can help us use our time more wisely and remind us to see the value in everyone and everything around us.

I will let others know I value them, and why.

September 22

It is only the strong who are strengthened by suffering; the weak are made weaker.

— *Lion Feuchtwanger*

In emergency health situations, people expect us to be a little more dependent and needy. But overly dependent behavior is not okay. We know it's not easy, when we are really suffering, to move to a position of strength, to create a new, mature attitude upon which we can base our behavior. It's difficult to unlearn old ways and to regroup our thoughts and actions. But using a ''sickie'' role is one of the behaviors we need to avoid.

Ultimately, no one is responsible for our mental and physical well-being but ourselves. As time goes by, we understand that we gain strength from our illness when we accept that responsibility.

My health difficulties can strengthen my attitude and my actions.

Physical courage, which despises all danger, will make a man brave in one way; and moral courage, which despises all opinion, will make a man brave in another. The former would seem most necessary for the camp; the latter for the council; but to constitute a great man, both are necessary.
— C. C. Colton

We are blessed to have many kinds of courage. We just never expected to have them all tested during a course of several years! Our physical courage increases every time we face a new situation or a different medical problem. Although we're not grateful for the illness itself, it has provided the challenges which have prompted greater courage in us. We've also had to look more closely at our values and had to become stronger in protecting them. We're more conscious of the choices we make and how we make them, and we're grateful for that awareness.

I will continue to make healthy, moral choices.

September 24

*To be what we are, and to become
what we are capable of becoming is
the only end of life.*
— *Robert Louis Stevenson*

Mountain climbers, river rafters, and marathon racers all face the "challenge of a lifetime." We have heard that phrase before, but may not have realized that our challenge of a lifetime would take a different form.

We all face challenges as we move through adulthood. In some instances — pain or illness, for example — we must face the obstacles placed in our way. We cannot choose to ignore or avoid them. One of our biggest challenges is the struggle to maintain a positive mental attitude. This is easier said than done when altered health patterns change lifestyles, but we can be on guard to think about "wellness" before "illness" and to remember we have been facing challenges all along.

I face challenges every day — some public, but many private. I will try to do my personal best.

Fate chooses our relatives. We choose our friends.

— *Jacques Bossuet*

We had no choice — and still have no choice — as to whether our families are supportive and caring. Those of us who lived in negative or unnurturing families may find that we slip into similar situations as adults. Without realizing it, we may have fostered friendships that allow us to use the same old scripts — the same unhealthy scripts.

One of the things we've learned from our illnesses is we must be willing to nurture ourselves. We need approval and love, and we have it within our power to give that gift to ourselves. We also can enter only into friendships based on these qualities, allowing us to be cared for and to care for others.

I choose today to work toward healthy, loving friendships.

September 26

*The modern sympathy with invalids
is morbid. Illness of any kind is hardly
a thing to be encouraged in others.*
— *Oscar Wilde*

When chronic illness strikes, there are
no rules of social behavior we can fall back
on. Nothing prepares us for the harsh
reality of illness. There is a very delicate
balance here. We want those who love us
to understand, and we want them to help,
but not to pity us.

We need to face squarely the changes
that chronic illness brings, both for our
loved ones and for us. By openly talking
to each other about our problems of adjustment and loss, we can become less preoccupied with our losses and think more
about the future. We will be less concerned with being ''in-valid.'' We can
move forth to a meaningful and valid life.

*Facing the changes caused by chronic illness can,
in the long run, serve to make me stronger.*

> *. . . We love persons . . . by reason of their defects as well as of their qualities.*
>
> *— Jacques Maritain*

There is a freedom in loving and being loved. The love we have for other special people frees us to concentrate on them, and we forget ourselves and our problems. Often, these people — our friends and family members — are loved by us not because we find perfection in them, but because we magically seem to blend together, and their faults become unimportant.

In being loved, we discover the same freedom. We don't have to conceal our defects. We can be open. Certainly, we continue to work to free ourselves of defects, but we do it for ourselves; we don't have to be perfect to deserve love. Nonjudgmental love is one of the things that frees us to make choices without fear.

I treasure all the loving friendships I have. They allow me to choose new directions by accepting me where I am.

September 28

A positive, responsible person does not forget the past harm which may have been done because of earlier ignorance, thoughtlessness, or emotional limitations.

— *Lewis F. Presnall*

We've learned to forgive those who we felt had done harm to us. Our pain diminished over time, and we were able to let go of our bad feelings.

We are much less accepting of our own errors. Years later we may continue to mercilessly judge ourselves for past mistakes. We can forgive ourselves by offering ourselves the same understanding we have offered those we love. As we move to a new, gentler way of looking at ourselves, we can accept the mistakes we've made in the past and even understand them in context of where we were at the time.

I can remember past mistakes I have made, but I will be gentle with myself when I see how far I have come.

Though we travel the world over to find the beautiful, we must carry it with us or we find it not.
— *Ralph Waldo Emerson*

Our culture encourages a quest for outer beauty, even though we know it is more important to have inner beauty. This is the beauty truly valued by others. We can live joyfully; we can delight in discovering and enjoying beauty. We are surrounded with loveliness in nature and in people's thoughts, words, and deeds. To accept that beauty, we must carry within ourselves a sensitivity, an appreciation for what is offered, and that sensitivity is a large part of the beauty we carry within us.

Life is full of beauty. I will keep my eyes open to the beauty that is in others, in nature, and in myself.

September 30

There is no failure except in no longer trying.
— *Elbert Hubbard*

It would be tragic to live our lives without direction, to never try to fulfill any dreams. Perhaps we have felt that we do not have direction in our lives any longer, or that we can't fulfill the lifelong dreams we had. By setting new goals and priorities in terms of today's reality, we can still have dreams and see them come true.

We might be tempted to resign ourselves to being failures, to set ourselves no new challenges, and to think of ourselves as victims. If we don't become fatigued with thoughts of resignation and failure, we will have the necessary energy to pursue new goals.

I am setting new goals that are realistic, and I will invest my energy in them.

October

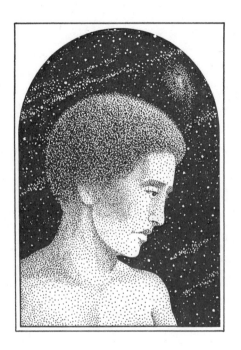

*Solitude is not measured by the miles
of space that intervene between a man
and his fellows.*
— *Henry David Thoreau*

Solitude is the time we choose to be alone, but it becomes loneliness when we believe we have no choice. When we are lonely, we feel trapped in a web of isolation.

Lonely people are caught in a trap with only themselves for company. There can be a difference between loneliness and aloneness — or solitude.

We are finding ways to create solitude from loneliness. We strive to fill our lives with meaningful experiences such as work, family, hobbies, and relationships with friends. As we enrich our lives with these activities, our alone time becomes solitude — a peaceful time to withdraw from the world and into thoughts, prayers, and meditation.

A moment of solitude today can enrich and replenish me.

October 2

God wrote His loveliest
poem on the day
He made the first tall, poplar tree,
And set it high upon a pale-gold hill
For all the now enchanted earth to see.
— Grace Noll

Autumn was such a wonderful time when we were youngsters. Raking meant gleefully jumping into mountains of leaves and later gathering with our families to watch the blazing piles.

We can still enjoy the trees and leaves around us. If we take time to observe even a single leaf, we will again be surprised at its beauty, its perfection. The golden or red or brown leaf is a small part of nature's balance.

We enjoyed trees before; we can find multiple ways to enjoy them now. Like all of the world around us, the leaves lend color, beauty, and meaning to our lives, if we only look.

All natural beauty deserves a second look before
I turn away.

Most of all, we seek to help them rise to what for most is the supreme challenge of their lives, by developing and enjoying their unique personalities to the fullest.

— Bernie S. Siegel

Just living life, not enjoying it, is a tread-water posture some of us adopt in our lives. Afraid to get ''too involved'' in living, we wait for the worst to occur. We look for a guide, a leader, to direct our path to physical and spiritual survival.

At first, we may be devastated when we realize that no one else can direct us, guide us, or lead us out of the maze of emotions that accompanies a chronic illness. Others can help, but only if we lead. Gradually we're finding a unique strength within us, one we'd not known before, that enables us to direct our physical and spiritual programs with greater confidence.

I am on a continuing journey to accept the challenges of my life. Allowing my unique personality to surface is the beginning.

October 4

The bitter and the sweet come from the outside, the hard from within, from one's own efforts.
— *Albert Einstein*

Too often we expect to have lives in which only happy events occur and no one is ever hurt. Instead of tears and sadness, we expect only happiness. In doing this, we do not face life realistically. By ignoring all the problems around us — our own and others' as well — we skim the surface of life.

When we face reality, we begin our real journey. A life well lived is not one of constant happiness and joy. More often, it is the life as lived by someone who has known intense pain and extreme disappointment. Our negative experiences give us that opportunity to be strengthened within.

All my experiences give me a chance to grow.

*Be patient with everyone, but above
all with yourself.*
— *St. Francis de Sales*

Like fine cheese, we wait, as we grow
older, to ripen properly. We would like to
hurry the process along, but haste won't
serve us well in the long run. We have
learned to let others take their time to mature and to become responsible adults, but
often when it comes to ourselves, we are
quick to anger at our own mistakes. We
frequently are not as forgiving of ourselves
as we are of others.

Maturity arrives when we understand
that some of the goals we thought were
crucial are really unattainable, and that it
really doesn't matter. Maturity is a frame
of mind where we learn to be pleased with
what we can accomplish. We can find
contentment in just living our days as best
we can.

*I recognize there is no magic moment when I
will become a fully mature adult. Maturity is an
attitude that conveys peace with myself.*

October 6

Every human being is a problem in search of a solution.
— *Ashley Montagu*

Despite the occasional distance or coolness that many of us sense within, we are also aware of wellsprings of emotion, ready to flow with feelings that have been long hidden. It sometimes takes a crisis, such as illness, chemical dependency, or loss of a loved one to literally drive us to seek help.

Trying to uncover deeply hidden painful emotions can feel like a treacherous path to follow, and some of us may be tempted to stop trying. But if we honestly open ourselves to these feelings, we can begin to know ourselves better and to build healthier and more mature relationships.

Change can be frightening, especially when I've been hiding from my own emotions. If there is a problem, dealing with my emotions is part of the solution.

Honor your challenges, for those spaces that you label as dark are actually there to bring you more light.
— *Sanaya Roman*

Many of us have wondered whether we should begin using adaptive living aids openly. We worry about what people would think if they saw us using equipment that brands us as handicapped. We fear embarrassment. Some folks never solve the problem, and they stay home, trapped by their fears of being noticed, of being different. It's difficult to forfeit the anonymity of being the same as everyone else.

One thing is certain — without special gadgets, we have to ask for help. So, with foresight and a fierce sense of independence, many of us grasp any opportunity to ''do'' for ourselves. We can use aids because they will assist and support our zest for life.

I will risk being different. By using adaptive devices I can remain more independent.

October 8

*Love is all we have, the only way that
each can help the other.*
— Euripides

We may tend to love our family members only with qualifications. Only if they don't complain about their problems. Only if they are more successful. Perhaps we don't say this directly, but we might be communicating these qualifications to our loved ones by holding back or by making indirect suggestions as to how they should live their lives.

We may be able to give our love more fully if we remember how much we need acceptance. We don't want to receive love that is prefaced by "only if . . . " Only if we don't complain. Only if we stop talking about our illness. We all need the comfort and support of love based on what we are, not on what others think we can or should be. Our loved ones need the same thing.

Knowing I am loved and can love others in an unqualified manner strengthens me.

*Bitterness and anger seem to be very
closely related and are interchangeable
words for the same emotion.*
— *Robert Lovering*

Bitterness and anger don't arrive out of
the blue when there is a health change.
Chronic illness doesn't cause these reactions, but it may bring these and other
feelings to light.

If negative emotions and attitudes cause
us pain or embarrassment, if we are unhappy with ourselves, it may be time to
take a personal inventory. How do we act
toward other people? What do we expect?
Do we create our own problems?

We can change negatives into positives,
but it requires time and great emotional
effort. Our attitudes do improve when
we want to change, when we're willing
to grow, and when we're patient with
ourselves.

*I can begin today to change my negative emo-
tions by admitting them and asking for the help
I need.*

October 10

> *But if a man happens to find himself
> . . . he has a mansion which he can
> inhabit with dignity all the days of his
> life.*
>
> — *James Michener*

If only, we think, I could regain that
joy, that feeling of being so pleased with
myself that I had as a child. If we think
about it, we might decide that the child
didn't disappear; it may still be waiting to
be freed once again.

We can pause and look at what we
have become as adults. If we seek self-
worth by pleasing or impressing others,
we may have stopped listening to that
childlike voice that tells us to trust ourselves. Dignity, self-worth, contentment
— these things grow out of a sense of self,
not from the opinions of others.

*The choices I make today will be based on my
own values.*

*Power said to the world, "You are
mine," The world kept it prisoner on
her throne. Love said to the world,
"I am thine." The world gave it the
freedom of her house.*
— *Rabindranath Tagore*

We all need to test our spiritual muscles. At first those muscles may seem
weak. It's natural after a lengthy bout with
illness to wonder why we were chosen for
pain, misery, or illness.

After a time, we become ready to learn
more about our own spirituality. We open
our minds and our hearts. As we explore this wonderful side of ourselves, we
discover our worth, our strengths, our
wholeness. And we discover that we are
not alone, that a Higher Power is sharing
His strength and peace with us.

*Today, I will learn more about my spirituality
than I knew yesterday. I will feel the peace and
strength given to me by my Higher Power.*

October 12

*Joy . . . is found only in the good
things of the soul.*

— *Philo*

Every day has its ups and downs — its
good and bad moments. The joys that today offers must be personally claimed, by
each of us, or they will pass by unnoticed.

The events that cause a joyful experience are different for all individuals. We
sometimes share joyful experiences with
other people. Watching an infant walk
for the first time can be a shared joy and
a lasting memory. Recognizing that our
friends, or perhaps even ourselves, have
found help in dealing with personal problems or harmful behaviors can also be joyful experiences.

Joy can also be a private time — fishing
on a lovely morning, watching the petals
of a flower unfold, or being part of a
growing relationship. All contribute to our
sense of well-being.

*In this day, I will be aware of the people and
activities that give me joy.*

You learn to build your roads on to-
day, because tomorrow's ground is too
uncertain for plans, and futures have
a way of falling down in mid-flight.
— *Veronica Shoffstal*

We may have lived a significant portion
of our adult lives planning for the future.
Although we must make some provision
for tomorrow — savings accounts, wills,
pension plans — our attempts to live a full,
rewarding life must be made each day.

Growth occurs in the present; it's never
accomplished if it's postponed until tomorrow. Each day we choose the direction
of our lives, whether we know it or not.
Either we take positive steps toward better goals and stronger values, or we move
not at all by ''planning'' our lives in some
uncertain future.

I will make good choices for myself in the reality
of today.

October 14

Nothing sharpens sight like envy.
　　　　　　　— Thomas Fuller

It's natural to want to own things — a house, a car, nice clothes, a boat. Once in a while we are able to save and buy some things we like, but more often we have to set priorities and choose which items really matter to us most.

Almost all of us know someone who *does* seem to have it all — materially — and we may be envious. Perhaps, at those times we can better serve our needs if we reexamine our values and cast our eyes toward other people who have the things we really want — peace of mind, a loving nature, spiritual depth, and an unjealous nature. Those ''things'' may be what we should strive to own. These qualities can be purchased only with time, and enrich our lives more than mere material objects ever could.

I will take inventory of my qualities, not my possessions.

*We cannot tear out a single page from
our life, but we can throw the whole
book into the fire.*
> — *George Sand*

During those darkest times, we may not
be able to think beyond this moment, this
pain, this loss. All we're aware of is this
tiny piece of time, and it casts its darkness
on all we remember and all we see in the
future.

This moment is a fraction of a lifetime;
this feeling is just one perception among
thousands we've experienced. We owe it
to ourselves to be sure of what we are
experiencing before discarding the entire
book in order to rid ourselves of one hated
page. If needed, we can explore our emotions with a professional. We can work
within a group of people who understand.
We can wait a while to see what our lives
will hold. We can look for change outside
and inside ourselves.

*My feelings are real, but so is the chance that
better things lie ahead. I pray for patience.*

October 16

Don't let life discourage you; everyone who got where he is had to begin where he was.
— *Richard L. Evans*

There's an old adage that good teachers still use: Start the child from where he is. In fact, we all have to begin from where we are. We may, at first, have a tendency to measure all our successes with our healthy life before our medical condition changed. Changed circumstances can play havoc with our lives.

Now we may have to set more realistic goals in order to reach them. We can still begin new jobs or new relationships. We begin over and over again throughout a lifetime — with or without a long-term medical situation. What matters most is how successfully we can handle the change. We'll do fine as long as we remember we have started anew many times — successfully.

I will not be discouraged by changes in my life. I have coped before, and I will again.

Maturity: among other things — not to hide one's strength out of fear and consequently live below one's best.
— *Dag Hammarskjold*

The fear of being different is a powerful force in our lives, especially in the early times after a chronic illness is diagnosed. We fear being recognized as a victim of an illness, and we become afraid of any recognition at all.

We don't want to live with this unreasonable fear, and we begin to understand that healthy thinking requires us to develop and use our many strengths. We stop denying and start accepting. The voice of our individuality begins to speak, loudly and clearly, and we answer with definitive action. We start to face our problems, to accept the ways in which we differ from others, and to rejoice in our strengths.

I won't hide my strengths, for they are the means to life at its best.

October 18

He that can't endure the bad, will not
live to see the good.
— *Yiddish Proverb*

Maturity means taking the bitter with
the sweet. Wisdom is the realization that
sometimes the two are interrelated. An
example of this is chronic illness. At first,
we might have been bitter because the
quality of our lives was changed.

Now, with a clearer perspective and
greater maturity, we realize that many
of the sweeter aspects of our lives today
have grown out of our learning to cope
with chronic illness. We live more in
the moment, rather than always pursuing
some distant goal. Our values reflect a
stronger sense of self; they emphasize
people over things. For many of us, the
growth, the joy, and the self-esteem that
now sweeten our lives come from the bitter
experiences of chronic illness.

I accept that my life experiences will be both good
and bad. Although my illness is unwanted, I
have been strengthened by it.

*There must be something strangely
sacred in salt. It is in our tears and
in the sea.*

— *Kahlil Gibran*

Emotion plays around a person's face,
making it strained or relaxed. We say we
can "read" someone else's face. Few of
us burst into spontaneous tears or laughter, but instead first show slight emotion
on our faces or in the way we speak.

Laughter is instrumental to our well-
being, but tears are also essential to our
emotional survival. When we finally release the emotions we feel and the dams
break loose, the tears are healing. They
allow us to cleanse ourselves of pent-up
angers, fears, and frustrations.

*I know crying is a human characteristic. I will
not be ashamed of my need to cry, for tears are
part of my human experience.*

October 20

*By a tranquil mind I mean nothing
else than a mind well ordered.*
— *Marcus Aurelius Antoninus*

When we are diagnosed as having a permanent medical condition, we may think we'll never know tranquility again. Before too long, though, we realize that whether we are entirely healthy or not, we bring to our new challenge the same value system we always had. We can still find peace and serenity in our lives, for we continue to live our lives as well as we are able.

We owe it to ourselves to search out tranquility — a state in which we feel extremely peaceful, at ease with our inner strength, with nature, and with our sense of higher purpose. Walking hand in hand with tranquility creates harmony, a time when our thoughts are orderly and we feel little distress.

I will work on keeping a peaceful mind in order to smooth out my rougher days.

*Business runs after nobody; people
cling to it of their own free will and
think that to be busy is a proof of
happiness.*
— *Lucius Annaeus Seneca*

Sometimes we need to keep busy just
to fill time. After a loss or health change,
we may have great amounts of time to fill.
We may turn to busy work — work having no significance but marking time as
we move toward yet another adjustment.
Tool-shop organizing, closet cleaning, and
other tasks might be ploys we need, emotionally, to perform in rote fashion.

When we are adjusting, we may need to
be busy — to think, to decide on new plans
of action, and to move forward. We won't
need busy work, and we'll be able to make
gains again. As we make our adjustments,
very, very slowly, the purpose of our lives
will return.

*I will put effort into my days to find meaning.
It may be difficult to stay busy, but I can do it.*

October 22

This is the bitterest knowledge among men, to have much knowledge but no power.

— *Herodotus*

We have the power to influence others' lives only when we share what we have learned. If we fail to or refuse to recognize the value of our knowledge, we force ourselves into a sort of isolation and — worse still — deprive others of our insights.

We know how to handle intricate personal relationships and delicate problems. We have gained the emotional stability to allow ourselves to depend on others and on our Higher Power. We can share this knowledge with others, not to serve our own needs, but to help our fellow human beings.

A loving power is mine when I gently share the knowledge I have with others.

*The more passionately we love life, the
more intensely we experience the joy
of life.*

— *Jurgen Moltman*

While we would occasionally like to hide
from the real-life drama around us, we
know it's not a healthy way to live. Instead
we live the drama, love it, cry with it, and
at times even hate it.

Choosing to live life on its terms brings
enthusiasm and passion into our experiences. Our decision to love life — despite
the highs and lows — allows us to delight
in the highs and to accept the lows as un-
avoidable, but momentary, setbacks. Although hiding from reality can sometimes
insulate us from pain, it also blinds us to
the joys and wonderment of living fully.

I choose to be enthusiastic about my life.

October 24

We conceal it from ourselves in vain
— we must always love something.
                              — Blaise Pascal

Not knowing how to love may imperil our very existence. Although love doesn't literally nourish our bodies, not being able to love strips us of our humanness.

Romantic love is only one part of our capacity to love, for there is also the ability to love our friends, family, and our fellow human beings. The ripple effect of our well-being will spread, both within us and from us, and we will begin to nourish our souls as well.

We also learn to love ourselves — all that we are. Self-love enhances our self-image. A strong sense of esteem enhances our entire lives.

I need to love and be loved. It is essential to my psychic well-being that I understand the importance of loving.

The more things you love, the more you are interested in, the more you enjoy, the more you have left when anything happens.
— *Ethel Barrymore*

Now is a good time for us to pursue our interests and to nurture both new and old relationships. We understand so well how easily and quickly our circumstances can change. This understanding nudges us to expand our experiences.

No one of us is immune from the troubles of life. Whether the problem is loss of a job or loss of a home, good health, or a dear friend, we all suffer at one time or another. Keeping our lives as full as possible with the love of good people and the challenge of activities provides support even when times get tough.

Tragedies and hard times will affect me, but I know I have the ability to move on.

October 26

Don't part with your illusions. When they are gone, you may still exist, but you have ceased to live.
— *Mark Twain*

Even as we approached young adulthood, we clung to our dreams about the future. In those days it may have seemed to us that anything was possible.

It's not immature to hold on to a dream, even when we know the dream is unlikely to come true. Bald men wish for a full head of hair. Some of us wish we still had young skin. Even though a long-term medical condition has become part of our lives, many of us still hold on to the illusions of our health being restored.

Now we have a few more years — or decades — behind us. We accept that some things are possible and some are not. Most of us are comfortable with that knowledge. And still we hope.

I hold dearly to many of my illusions. The possibilities of what might occur keep my days full of excitement.

Better be alone than in bad company.
— *Thomas Fuller*

Most of us have had the experience of being befriended by someone who seems to want to spend every waking moment in our company. At first, we may be delighted with the attention and enjoy the excitement of the developing relationship. Then, suddenly we feel smothered. The other person gives us no time alone; he or she is such a constant presence that we feel out of touch with ourselves.

We seem to have to choose between crushing our new friend or submitting to the constant intrusion, but first we may need to remind ourselves that we have the right to create the framework of our days. If bad company or just constant company is not our choice, we are free to say, ''I need more time alone.'' This isn't a rejection of others; it's an affirmation of ourselves and our need for solitude.

I can find a healthy balance between my time with others and my time alone.

October 28

Yesterday is not ours to recover, but
tomorrow is ours to win or lose.
— *Lyndon B. Johnson*

We can cherish our yesterdays or even regret them, but we can never live them again. The past is behind us; the future lies ahead. We may sometimes be saddened by the thought that the future might be shorter than our past, but we find comfort in remembering that the future is real and promising; the past is neither.

To find only positives in the past and negatives in the future robs us of one of our greatest gifts — time — and time is what the past can't give us. Yesterday's gifts to us are memories, and an occasional backward glance to what once was is natural. But we grow mentally and spiritually by living in this day and planning for tomorrow.

I accept the gifts of yesterday's memories, today's reality, and tomorrow's dreams.

You may talk on all subjects save one,
namely, your maladies.
> — *Ralph Waldo Emerson*

Casual conversations have an unspoken rule: never, never tell about our pain, our misery, our difficulties. Ironically, the stars of social gatherings are often the ones who have just suffered an accident or injury. We show interest and concern for new and obvious problems; we often ignore ongoing ones. A leg cast has glamor; a wheelchair has none.

We can understand this. Human nature finds adventure in broken bones or neck braces. It also finds reassurance because these injuries are temporary and the victim will be as good as new in a matter of weeks. Many people can't identify with the permanence of chronic illness, but we can educate them about our social concerns without provoking pity.

My life becomes more balanced when I enjoy social activities as social — not medical — events.

October 30

*We can have a hand in our own daily
miracle of health.*
              — Lewis F. Presnall

Some things we cannot change or control, and one of those most certainly is the limiting nature of illnesses. But we're not alone. We have surely learned by now that all people have to deal with handicaps or limitations — physical, psychological, or emotional. Like all other people, we are challenged to live a fulfilling life within the limitations placed upon us.

What matters most is that even though we may have a long-term health problem, we can learn to dwell on wellness, not on illness. Limitations certainly affect how we live our lives, but they need not alter the quality of who we are. It's up to us to choose whether we will be all we are intended to be.

There are large areas which I can still control in my life, and that gives me hope.

*The human body is the best picture of
the human soul.*
— *Ludwig Wittgenstein*

As people walk down the street, we can usually spot those with a sense of pride in themselves. How people look is often an indicator of their self-esteem. The changes in our lives challenge us to continue feeling good about ourselves despite stress or diminished health. Any change can be frightening. Unfortunately, sometimes we let problems overtake us, and we begin to look and act like people who feel unwell.

We can take stock of our lives at this time and remember how much we can still do well. We are capable individuals; we can make our own decisions about how we want to conduct our lives. This renewed awareness strengthens our self-esteem, and the image we convey to others is one of pride.

*There are some things I just cannot change.
Today, I will dwell on what I can do for myself.*

November

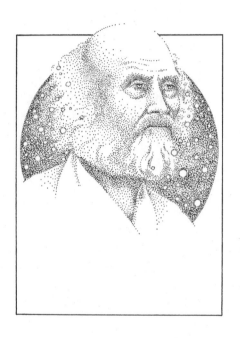

*Old age, to the unlearned, is winter;
to the learned, it is harvest time.*
— *Judah Leib Lazerov*

Too many of us fear old age, for it is seen all too often as merely the bridge between retirement and senility or death. This, of course, is only a myth. Advancing years do not automatically mean poor health or dependency.

We should always be aware of the pride and integrity that come with old age. Some older people stand as role models to youth. Decades of work have honed skills which can and should continue to be used in various ways. There is always more to learn and more to do. We can use our time to pursue interests and to develop any skills that give us joy.

I will not be frightened of growing older, for I intend to do so with the pride and integrity developed with age and experience.

November 2

Grace is the absence of everything that indicates pain or difficulty, hesitation or incongruity.
— William Hazlitt

Grace is the power to look within ourselves and become stronger. When we're truly gracious, we try to put ourselves in another's place so we can imagine how that person might feel. This becomes an especially important issue when we are physically impaired, for those around us will take their cue from our behavior.

Trying to cope with the internal forces of health changes can be very lonely. When we need to use assistive devices such as canes, walkers, or wheelchairs, other people may at first not know quite how to react. We can help ease their discomfort and guide their reactions by our positive actions.

I will be gracious to others by being aware of their level of comfort when we are together.

It is well to give when asked, but it is better to give when unasked through understanding.

— Kahlil Gibran

Some of us wonder how we will live the rest of our lives with the problems we are currently carrying. The days loom long, with no specific goals in sight; so it is up to us to formulate new plans and goals for ourselves.

These plans — social, spiritual, academic, or volunteer — are good for us if they revolve around other people, many of whom have even greater problems than ours. Sharing our hope, faith, and varied experiences with others who also suffer is a caring gesture and an opportunity to see ourselves and our problems more clearly within the total human picture.

Today, I will choose some way to help myself and others. Sharing my experiences and skills keeps me in touch with my humanness.

November 4

You cannot create experience. You must undergo it.
— *Albert Camus*

Who among us hasn't wanted to play with or read to a pleading child? Who hasn't thought of volunteering some time so others — and we — could have happier and richer lives? We may have put off or refused these opportunities because we felt overwhelmed by the limitations of a chronic illness. Perhaps we felt like victims who had lost an essential power to control our lives.

Our days are increasingly better when we understand that all experience, good and bad, isn't orchestrated by us — and it never was. Yet this doesn't mean we are helpless. We now see choices and chances to let our actions be positive life-affirming statements. We see opportunities for sharing, for joining in, and for reaching out. And we take them.

I will concentrate on making good choices, not just easy choices.

*I remember those happy days and of-
ten wish I could speak into the ears of
the dead the gratitude which was due
to them in life and so ill-returned.*
— *Gwyn Thomas*

We respond to loss in predictable ways.
One common response to loss — whether
of a loved one or of good health — is
regret. ''I should have told him how
much he was loved,'' or ''I wish I'd told
her I was sorry for what I said.'' These
statements of regret are much like the
regrets accompanying chronic illness. ''I
wish I'd pursued my dreams when I was
healthy.'' We move out of our sadness
only when we are able to remember that
our only mistake was a human one —
always believing there would be more time
to say and do the things we wanted. Our
healing is complete when we bring this
awareness to the present, when we say and
do positive things today.

*Letting go of past regrets frees me to be a more
loving person today.*

November 6

*To achieve great things we must live
as though we were never going to die.*
— *Vauvenarques*

Of all the limitations we face, one of the greatest is actually one we impose upon ourselves. We limit ourselves by believing that it's too late to go back to school, to change careers, or to start something new. We artificially restrict ourselves because we misunderstand the concept of time.

We can decide if time is a friend or an enemy. It's our enemy when we shy away from new experiences. But when we willingly take unsteady steps into unknown territory by lifting a brush to canvas or finally learning to drive a car or applying for the job we've always wanted, then time is our friend. We have all the time in the world because we have *this* moment, this day, and that is all the time we need to begin great things.

I am the only one who can decide which great things I will begin today.

*Night brings our troubles to the light,
rather than banishes them.*
— Lucius Annaeus Seneca

One of our greatest coping skills is setting realistic expectations. In doing so, we're less likely to moan and complain. We're not so filled with self-pity. We are learning to use all our resources when we lie awake struggling with physical or emotional pain.

We can help ourselves by making our bedroom surroundings as pleasant as possible. Adding small items, such as flowers, bookcases, and a mini-reading lamp isn't just a cosmetic improvement. It's admitting that we might be spending some wakeful time in there. Some nights might be sleepless, but admitting it and preparing for it may make the experience less frightening and more restful.

If I can't sleep, I can relax in the comfort of my bedroom.

November 8

> *We often experience more regret over*
> *the part we have left, than pleasure*
> *over the part we have preferred.*
> — *Joseph Roux*

We may sometimes think about past loves, jobs we turned down, or educations we didn't pursue. This nostalgic inventory may give us more regret than joy.

A more accurate picture of our lives is found in the things we've chosen. We can start with the communities in which we live. Quickly, we find ourselves listing such intangibles as spiritual experiences, family times of togetherness, friendships, and love. Seeing life more clearly as a balance between mistakes and triumphs, disappointments and joys, can encourage us to expect the same balance each day.

I have less regret for what I've lost when I focus on the many good things I've chosen.

Faith is a living and unshakeable con-
fidence, a belief in the grace of God so
assured that a man would die a thou-
sand deaths for its sake.
                              — Martin Luther

When a crisis ocurs — a death in the family or perhaps a chronic illness — many of us pass through the ''Why me?'' phase. We may become confused and feel we have been personally selected for bad times. Our faith may be shaken. It can take us a while to recognize that we still have abiding faith in our Higher Power. Time passes and as life gains some semblance of normalcy again, we understand there are no easy answers, but our faith has carried us through a difficult time.

Eventually, our belief in a Power greater than ourselves takes hold, rather firmly, until we feel an even stronger sense of faith and purpose than before.

As I gain my own strengths I am more able to extend my beliefs to include my Higher Power once again.

November 10

It is easier to confess a defect than to claim a quality.
— *Max Beerbohm*

It is easy to simply admit our character defects — and then do nothing about them. The difficult part is asking God — however we picture God — to remove our defects and then live with the choices we have made.

We may have apologized to friends, and then added, "but I've always been that way." Or, "I just can't seem to help it." We might have used such excuses to avoid looking honestly at ourselves. When we sincerely examine our character defects and have the desire to change, our confessions to others no longer are made with excuses. Instead, we admit our flaws, ask our Higher Power to remove them, and then take responsibility for working toward qualities we admire.

My defects can be changed once I admit them and begin to work on eliminating them.

*Pray that your loneliness may spur
you into finding something to live for,
great enough to die for.*
— *Dag Hammarskjold*

The first time we go through a festive season without our spouse or a dear friend or beloved child, we may wonder if we can get through it. Pity overwhelms us as we think, Surely no one has felt as bad as I do right now. Pain increases our loneliness, and we feel crushed by the holiday preparations the rest of the world seems to be making.

We can struggle out of this self-imposed misery by using the strategies that have helped us cope with our chronic illnesses. Patience tells us that this too shall pass. Selflessness shows us others who need compassion more than we do. Spirituality reminds us that our pain and sadness can be entrusted to the loving care of our Higher Power.

I know the holidays can be difficult, and if I take them one day at a time I will do just fine.

November 12

Life is the enjoyment of emotion, de-rived from the past and aimed at the future.
— *Alfred, Lord Whitehead*

Life sails by much more quickly than we expect it to. When our children were young, it seemed as though endless years stretched ahead for us to nurture and teach them; suddenly they are in college, or married with children of their own.

Each day must be lived to its fullest, for we shall never be able to recapture it again. The memories we create today can enrich the present, and even future years. Making good memories serves us well.

It is our wish to fully enjoy life and, if we can't, to attempt to correct those prob-lems which keep us from fully enjoying what we do have. Then we can once again look to a full and wonderful future.

I will work to deal with those facets of my life which cause me pain.

Meditation is not a means to an end.
It is both the means and the end.
             — Krishnamurti

There is a current trend toward reading meditation books, which we're familiar with. We tend to use meditations as enlarged thoughts for the day. Some of us begin our days with a meditation; others of us use them as a final thought before bed.

Meditation encourages deep and comforting thoughts. How we meditate has little importance, for customs are different across the cultures. What does matter is that we are turning to rich spiritual resources, so that each day we can give some serious time to our most pertinent thoughts and to improving ourselves.

When I meditate I have a special thought to carry with me throughout the day. I know I am doing something important for myself.

November 14

Rest is not a matter of doing absolutely nothing. Rest is repair.
— *Daniel W. Josselyn*

Every once in a while the burdens of our lives get us down. We just can't be optimistic all the time. It's so important to know that we can let go of those burdens for a day or two; in fact, we owe it to ourselves.

Too many of us feel guilty if we succumb to our feelings of sadness, disgust, anger, or exhaustion. Why? Having a medical problem doesn't make us any more or less exempt from the problems which face everybody else. There will be days when there seems to be no reason to get out of bed. That's okay. We can take a mental health day by relaxing. We can pamper ourselves every once in a while to rejuvenate the physical and emotional strength needed to face our world.

I can simplify my life by giving myself this day for relaxing.

*There is always room for improve-
ment, you know — it's the biggest
room in the house.*
— *Louise Heath Leber*

Accepting criticism is very hard, even
when it's given constructively. As small
children we may have bristled at suggestions about our drawings or toy houses we
made. We liked things to be the way we
wanted them to be.

Not everyone is so talented and sensitive
that they can offer criticism without it
hurting. We do ourselves justice when
we learn to listen to most criticism. Of
course, we retain the right to disagree.

We understand that criticism is often
tempered with love and understanding. A
receptiveness to criticism helps us become
less rigid and more willing to change.

*I can accept criticism and try to change when it
will benefit me.*

November 16

The future is an opaque mirror. Anyone who tries to look into it sees nothing but the dim outlines of an old and worried face.

— Jim Bishop

Perhaps we spend too much time looking into mirrors and being critical of what we see. There is no stage in life when we are wholly contented with what we see, but as we mature we gradually recognize that our lives are multidimensional. Now we know that there will be periods of time when we are more pensive, more introspective — and times when life will just roll along, with no concern from us.

Acceptance of our appearance gives us the time and energy to work on our inner selves. We look to the future by trying to prepare, and we live in the present by understanding that what we look like is not as important as what we do.

Today, I will decide which changes can give me and others the most joy.

The people plan, and God laughs.
— *Yiddish Proverb*

Through the ages our ancestors have recognized that sometimes what happens is due to a purely random selection. Natural disasters occur, accidents happen, and people are in the wrong places at the wrong times.

But what about being in the right place at the right time? It's not very often that we hear those stories. We hear about tragedies and real triumphs. What we don't hear are stories about people like us, who struggle along, doing the best they can, hoping for a break. We have learned there are times to let go of unrealistic plans and to let our Higher Power have a hand in our lives. By letting go we create our own well-being.

I make my plans and hope for success, knowing there is a Power greater than me who has the final word.

November 18

Life is not a static thing.
— *Everett M. Dirkson*

Sometimes change occurs so slowly within us that we don't notice it. We accept it and may even welcome it when it happens gradually, but we're less likely to accept those changes that arrive suddenly. Abrupt change doesn't fit what we expect and can cause chaos in our lives.

When we finally realize we can't prevent changes from happening, but can only alter our reactions to these changes, they become easier to accept. We can't stop our declining health either, but we can certainly understand the influence a positive attitude can have on our lives.

I will accept the things I cannot change.

There is no formula for easy living.
Anyone who says he has one is either
joking or lying.
— *Harold Russell*

We all have, in our mind's eye, a picture of what life would be like if we were healthy and wealthy and could do whatever we wanted with our days. If given the choice between health and sickness, wealth and poverty, most people would choose the former of both. Yet, there are no assurances of easy living no matter how healthy or wealthy we are.

When our wish to "have it easy" becomes a preoccupation — like living with severe pain — our whole system can become stressed. We need to recognize that this wish for "having it easy" creates stress that we could avoid. Ironically, to escape this stress, we need to return to the reality of our own beautiful lives.

I have no guarantee for easy living, but I am guaranteed the chance to change and grow as often as I want to.

November 20

There is no hope unmingled with fear,
and no fear unmingled with hope.
— *Baruch Spinoza*

Most of us are frightened each time we go through a major life change, for we fear what we do not know. We thought we had our lives planned. Because a crisis occurs unexpectedly, there is no way to prepare for a burglary, a broken leg, or loss of a loved one. These events can throw us and our lives into a tailspin.

If the event is short-lived, like a bad case of the flu or a minor injury, we forget it quickly. If, however, the effects are long-lasting, we work to incorporate them into our daily living. Adapting in this way forces us to look for the positive parts of the day. We get into the habit of remembering good times and hope — even expect — better times will come.

I can see that positive action and thought is needed. I will find good people and events in this day.

*To most of us the real life is the life
we do not lead.*

— *Oscar Wilde*

We don't enjoy feeling envious, but
there are times when we find ourselves
wishing we had what others do. "I
wish my body could do what hers does."
"I wish I didn't have to take all this
medicine. He doesn't have to."

After feeling envious, we need to return
to our own lives with enthusiasm. While
we may not be able to do what others do or
have what others have, our lives are filled
with experiences that can make us rich and
able people. Regardless of who we are,
what we own, or how we live, each of us
is living a very important life — complete
with pain, memories, and pleasure.

*I respect myself and this life I am living. Today,
I will concentrate on its joys and treasures.*

November 22

Just pray for a thick skin and a tender heart.

— *Ruth Graham*

There are times when we become angry or hurt or disappointed by the words or actions of our friends. When we react in any of these ways, we are focusing on them instead of us. "He hurt my feelings," we might say, or "She made me angry." These statements point out the error in our reasoning. No one can "make" us feel a certain way.

Our lives are happier and our emotions more even when we realize we are choosing our reactions. "I let myself be angry (or hurt or disappointed)." Knowing this, gives us a choice in how we let others affect us. We can be less sensitive to real or imagined wrongs. Instead, we can use our sensitivity to understand the pain of others.

I will be more loving toward my friends by overlooking their flaws and underlining their strengths.

*What's a man's first duty? The
answer is brief: To be himself.*
— *Henrik Ibsen*

We may tend to neglect ourselves, not
just physically, but emotionally and spiritually as well. We are generally aware
of what we're doing when we don't eat
right or get enough sleep, but we often are
blind to our neglect of inner needs. Each
of us needs privacy, to think, to plan, to
be away from the everyday clamor of our
lives.

We can take time for ourselves, even if
it's just a brief moment now and then. So
we can assess our life. So we can relax,
alone. So we can pray. So we can be
ourselves.

*I will not hide from myself under the guise of
being too busy. I can take time, just for myself,
to be aware of my personal needs.*

November 24

Kindness in words creates confidence.
Kindness in thinking creates
profoundness.
Kindness in giving creates love.
— *Lao Tzu*

As the holiday season approaches, we watch young families being swept up with the joy of the holiday season. It's natural to feel some self-pity, for it seems as though no holiday will ever be the same as the ones gone by.

Now it's time to make new memories. We can create them for ourselves. Who but ourselves do we have to blame for not having a good time at the holidays? Envying other people and the joy they share will serve no one. Have we shared with anyone today? Aren't there people who can be touched by our kind thoughts or actions? Can't we give of ourselves unselfishly? The holiday season is not about isolation; it is about reaching out.

I have the ability to bring old and new holiday traditions to others.

*Be a football to Time and Chance,
the more kicks the better, so that you
inspect the whole game and know its
utmost law.*
— *Ralph Waldo Emerson*

There's something attractive about living a controlled life, a life in which we're never embarrassed or disappointed or foolish. Perhaps it's safety we seek when we try to control everyone and everything around us. As is so often true, we can't get one thing without forfeiting another. In this case, if we choose safety, we lose spontaneity and excitement.

Although we don't want to take dangerous risks or make foolish choices when clearly better ones present themselves, we may want to loosen our tight, controlling grasp on our lives. To live fully and joyously, we do want and need to examine the range of experiences life offers. Yes, we may get a few bumps and bruises, but we'll also find joy and contentment.

Today, I will welcome the unexpected in my life.

November 26

*Trees and fields tell me nothing; men
are my teachers.*

        — *Plato*

Our earliest teachers were our parents,
and from them, if we were lucky, we
learned unqualified love and acceptance
and developed our religious beliefs. Later,
trained professionals taught us specific
subject matter. We also learned ethics
from our instructors, our parents, and our
house of worship.

A few of us may take issue with ''trees
and fields tell me nothing.'' But then we
realize that our appreciation of nature's
beauty was really taught and encouraged
by our parents and teachers. We observe
the glory of nature happening right before our eyes, but our understanding of
life, growth, and death comes from our
understanding of the teachings of people.

*I will keep my mind open to learn so that I can
make as many gains in learning as are available
to me.*

Bitterness imprisons life;
love releases it.
— *Harry Emerson Fosdick*

We sometimes waste far too much energy licking old wounds, nursing old hurts. Harboring bitterness only causes us pain. It folds all our feelings into a tight little package and keeps them hidden from sight.

Moving from bitter to loving feelings doesn't happen overnight, but it does happen when we nurture ourselves and open ourselves to others. Letting friends and family help is one way to begin. Soon we will remember how wonderful and unthreatening love feels. Outgoing, warm, and trusting feelings flow through us toward others. We can harness our love and use it for emotional recovery. Eventually, we are freed of unnecessary pain. We are learning once again to love in an unqualified way — and to love ourselves.

I do not need to be imprisoned by bitterness. I can set myself free.

November 28

Time deals gently only with those who take it gently.
— *Anatole France*

There have been times when we've taken our lives too seriously. For whatever reasons — family problems, money problems, health problems — we've let those concerns distort all the events of the day into sad or personally threatening experiences. When we've been preoccupied with negative thoughts, it's probably been difficult to see good possibilities.

Life magically becomes better, easier, when we take it gently in manageable segments. Problems may seem insurmountable if we insist on seeing them stretch into the coming months or years. But when we challenge ourselves to live in this day, the time treats us more gently by giving us a clearer picture of what we must deal with in this smaller segment of time.

Today, I will concentrate only on the things that must be dealt with in these twenty-four hours.

You should not hold back from making a start because of fears about the future.

— *Lewis F. Presnall*

Too often we fold up our dreams and set them aside because we can't envision success. The dream of a new business or of a new home or even of a self-improvement plan is easily discarded if we allow ourselves to think only of reasons why it won't work. Not enough money, we decide. Or, I don't have enough experience. Or — worse yet — I won't succeed because I never have before.

We can become free to pursue our dreams when we realize that the future is not an enemy waiting to thwart our efforts. What our tomorrows hold quite often depends on the decisions and moves we make today. Right now, we can make a start. We can set aside — not our dreams — but our fears of an unfriendly future.

The choices I make today will affect the quality of my future.

November 30

It is in vain to say human beings ought to be satisfied with tranquility: they must have action; and they will make it if they cannot find it.
— *Charlotte Bronte*

Tranquil: free from agitation; calm, peaceful. This we understand; this we desire. We surely want to have tranquil lives. Before chronic illness, we may have taken peace and tranquility for granted, for we were actively involved with the pursuit of life. Happiness and contentment came automatically along with the rest, with no conscious thought about it.

Before long we began to understand that if we wished to be tranquil, our minds and our bodies needed activity. Tranquility, that inner sense of calm, comes from contentment with how we are living our lives — and how actively we are living.

Tranquility will increase with my activity.

December

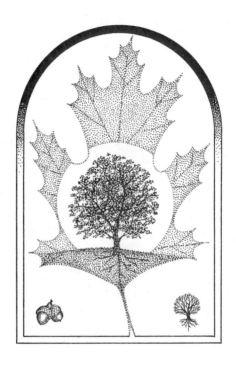

The wise man looks at death with honesty, dignity and calm, recognizing that the tragedy it brings is inherent in the great gift of life.
— *Corliss Lamont*

Chronic illness tends to heighten our awareness of the fragility of life. Some of us may even become concerned that due to poor health we may not live as long as we'd once expected.

To ease our fears, we may feel better if we initiated a conversation with family members about dying. Since each one of us has personal ideas about how we would like our funeral handled — which hymns, who will say the eulogy, and where it should be held — it only makes sense to share that information with loved ones. Few people feel comfortable talking about the possibility of dying, but with a straightforward discussion we can, at least for a while, set aside our own anxieties.

I am comforted knowing my family understands my fears and needs.

December 2

> *Habituation is a falling asleep or fatiguing of the sense of time; which explains why young years pass slowly, while later life flings itself faster and faster upon its course.*
> — Thomas Mann

Our routines can become so rote that we're unaware of making choices. Suddenly, we realize we haven't done many of the things which matter most to us. With this realization comes another: sometimes making no choice is, in fact, a choice in itself. If we move through each day doing the same things, saying the same words, living a copy of the day before — we have chosen to live safely. But we may think, I wish I had . . .

We don't have to completely change our lives in order to make better choices for ourselves. All we have to do is see all the choices open to us.

What and how I choose makes every day different from the last.

*Happiness is not being pained in body
nor troubled in mind.*
— *Thomas Jefferson*

Teenagers say it all the time: ''Hey!
Mellow out! Hype down!'' These words
may be alien to us, but we can listen to
these somewhat flippant admonitions.

Perhaps we do get too tense at times
during certain phases of our lives. Pain,
anxiety, or stress can cause us to tighten
our muscles, to brace our bodies against
the impact of our medical problems. The
tighter our bodies become, the less patient
and kind we are to those we love.

To help ourselves ''mellow out'' we
first have to identify the feelings associated with tenseness. We can calm down
by taking deep, slow, cleansing breaths.
Let's do ourselves a favor and learn to relax, to mellow out.

*By learning to let my body rest and relax, I
can concentrate on keeping my mind free and
untroubled.*

December 4

A tragedy means always a man's struggles with that which is stronger than man.

— G. K. Chesteron

Once the diagnosis of a long-term illness is learned, some of us may use it as an excuse to be sad, morbid, sullen, unfeeling, and uncaring. These behaviors are all counterproductive to the fulfilling life we want to lead.

Those of us who undergo a major health change may consider it a tragedy. It is; loss of good health is a frightening change. But to keep our personal problems hidden, to never reach out for help and for support — that is the truest tragedy.

We can reach out to those who love us and extend our arms to our Higher Power. Rather than being bitter, we can involve ourselves in the lives of others and allow our personal tragedies to generate triumphs.

My faith in a Higher Power and my faith in myself grow stronger each day.

*Forgiveness is the answer to the
child's dream of a miracle by which
what is broken is made whole again,
what is soiled is again made clean.*
— Dag Hammarskjold

We all may feel a measure of guilt when
relationships deteriorate or friends become
angry with each other. Sometimes, it's not
the people around us who are to blame;
sometimes it really is our fault. We've
misspoken or said harsh and unfeeling
words to a friend.

We can't undo our mistakes or take
back our words, but we can ask for forgiveness and try to make amends. We
can forgive others when they have hurt us,
knowing that forgiveness keeps our relationships whole.

*I don't have to wait for forgiveness from others;
I can make my amends first.*

December 6

A leader is a dealer in hope.
— *Napoleon Bonaparte*

A good leader doesn't always have the firmest hand or the most knowledge about a subject, but instead has the ability to develop hope and enthusiasm for success in others. Leading others often means being a role model; it means confidently marching forward, not pushing others from behind.

We all are leaders at one time or another. Raising children or working with others or nurturing relationships — all require leadership at times. Our health care also requires our leadership, and we find the most success when we lead with a hopeful spirit. That hope is reflected in our cooperation with the medical community, and it is also shown in our eagerness to live life fully and joyfully.

My hope, enthusiasm, and growth help me and others deal with chronic illness.

*Man adjusts to what he should not; he
is unable to adjust to what he should.*
— *Jean Toomer*

Most teenagers love French fries, pop,
and candy bars. We know that most fast-
food and sugar is bad for us — and so do
teenagers — but many of us continue to
munch on junk food.

Now that we have an adult's perspective, one would think that adjusting to
new things or getting rid of bad habits
would become easier. Not so! Adjusting
to change is not easy, particularly when it
involves our health.

One of the most difficult problems is
maintaining a balance between dealing
with the chronic problem and wanting to
live without it. We learn, despite our resistance to change, that we can have an
illness and can adjust — we can remain
strong and happy.

*I am confident of my ability to deal with my
illness, and live a good life.*

December 8

*There are some remedies worse than
the disease.*

— *Publilius Syrus*

Sometimes the very medicines prescribed to help us return to a more stable health situation can cause side effects
which can be nearly intolerable. How ludi-
crous that a drug intended to help us shake
off the exhaustion caused by a chronic
health condition can cause fatigue. What
a joke on us that a pill taken for arthritis, for example, can cause other potential
medical problems.

Despite these side effects, we should not
stop following dosage instructions until
we talk with our doctors, who can help
minimize the side effects. In this way we
will gain one more foothold in the process
of learning to live with our problems.

*I'll try to keep communication lines open with
my doctor to make it as easy as possible upon
myself.*

*To see the goal of life as "winning"
forces us to see other people as com-
petitors, threats to our happiness. For
us to "win," they have to "lose."*
— *Harold Kushner*

Our thinking is healthier when we see
our goals as individual accomplishments,
not as outdoing someone else. Others
don't have to get less or be less in order
for us to feel good about ourselves.

Rather than, "I beat someone out of a
job," we need to understand that it's not
a contest, but a matter of placing the most
qualified person in a new position. We all
have different skills, and it is usually the
skill, not the person, that is recognized
or rewarded. The person who possesses
the needed skill is not necessarily better,
nicer, or more worthwhile — even when
that person is us. In accepting that, we are
better able to work toward our personal
goals without fear of competition.

The only winning I pursue is meeting my goals.

December 10

In these times one must write with one's life. This is the challenge to all of us.
— *Antoine de St. Exupery*

When we were younger, many of us had a prescribed course of life — first school, a job, marriage, and then children. We never realized, and luckily so, that we would be dealt cards in a game we wouldn't want to play.

With the illnesses, sorrows, and pain have come joy, delight, and happiness. We would not have wanted to see into the future, but now that we are here, we all want to live life as well as we are able. The need to deal as best we can with our burdens advances us toward positive actions and thoughts. What good or bad things happen to us do not determine a life's story as much as the choices we make. We can choose to be challenged. We can choose our directions.

Changes or improvements can begin today with the decisions I make.

I've heard He works with broken people. I am sick, hurting, broken. I am waiting and willing now. . . .
— *Flora E. Meredith*

Sometimes life can feel so hopeless. Pain, anxiety about health, and fear can plague our thoughts. Admitting things are out of our control can be so hard. It takes a tremendous amount of courage to admit that we need help. Giving ourselves over to the care of our Higher Power is frightening when we have become used to taking care of our own needs.

The hardest job is ours, though, for we must be willing to let go of that part of ourselves that is troubled, in order to become whole once again. We must be willing to let go in order to be helped.

I have made the hardest move and placed myself into the care of my Higher Power. Now I must wait.

December 12

Unreal is action without discipline, charity without sympathy, ritual without devotion.

— Bhagavadgita

It's so easy to routinely go about our lives without examining our motives, without deciding why we do the things we do. We may have become so accustomed to reacting to what we think is expected of us that we rarely ponder what we expect of ourselves. At what point do we become willing to know ourselves?

Now may be the right moment to decide whether we act upon our own values, beliefs, and feelings, or whether we react to some vague sense of what others expect. By doing this, we might be surprised to discover that our charitable and spiritual actions do not change but they will become real because they are created by our inward sense of direction, discipline, love of others, and acceptance of self.

The things I say and do today will be directed by what I expect of myself, not by what I think others expect of me.

*'Tis a lesson you should heed, Try, try
again. If at first you don't succeed,
Try, try again.*
— *William E. Hickson*

Our teachers told us to try again. Our
parents reminded us to try again. And
sometimes we even did try again! Usually
it was something simple, like recopying
poorly written homework. We hardly realized then that we would be carrying that
message with us into adulthood. It's often
difficult to listen to good advice; it's even
harder to accept it.

When we learn to reassess our goals, to
reset priorities, and to be more realistic
about where we are really headed, trying
again begins to make more sense. Trying
again doesn't always mean doing it over
again. It can mean trying something entirely new. It can mean daring to change.

Trying again means I give myself room to grow.

December 14

I am just a heartbeat away from loneliness.

— *Laura Palmer*

The holiday season can be difficult for anyone who has had a major life change. A person who has been widowed, has moved, or has had to deal with new physical limitations may become lonesome when each holiday, birthday, or anniversary rolls around.

We sometimes cause ourselves pain by isolating ourselves. We may feel that no one wants to share the holiday with us or that we don't wish to impose the inconvenience of illness upon friends.

By reminding ourselves of the meaning of these special days, we often find that we can move out of our isolation. Holidays and other occasions reaffirm the value of tradition, love, and family. These days compel us to remember our place within a welcoming circle of friends and family.

I can choose to reach out during the holidays — or any day.

*The greatest of faults, I should say, is
to be conscious of none.*
— *Thomas Carlyle*

We really know that we are not perfect.
We are, like everyone else, beings capable of millions of behaviors. We can develop a humble self-awareness that takes
all of our pluses and minuses into account.
When we examine ourselves gently, but
honestly, we find ourselves in a position
where we can correct our own faults and
become more tolerant and accepting of the
faults of others.

The unconditional love we give ourselves — and everyone we care for — isn't
blind to imperfections; instead, it openly
accepts strengths and weaknesses.

*Today, my love of myself and others will be
shown in my tolerance of imperfections.*

December 16

*It is well that there is no one without
a fault, for he would not have a friend
in the world.*

— *William Hazlitt*

As youngsters we may have had doubts,
just as we do now, about making new
friends. We imposed unwritten rules upon
ourselves as we sought out new friends.
Will they like me? How do I approach
them? Will we have enough to talk about?

These questions are again in our minds
as we approach old and new relationships.
We might worry that since we aren't always feeling happy and well, our friends
might no longer value our company. This
is not usually true, but it may take us a
little while to pull away from fear and self-
doubt and to make real efforts at making
and maintaining our friendships.

*Today, I will let my friends know just how
important they are to me.*

Sadness flies on the wings of the morning and out of the heart of darkness comes the light.
— *Jean Giraudoux*

Many people — not just the chronically ill — experience a sense of sadness or longing at this time of year. Perhaps the season stirs memories of carefree, happier times or, instead, of holidays long ago that were unhappy and without fantasy.

Knowing that this sadness is not uncommon can be comforting and so is knowing we can resist sadness. If we're unhappy with old traditions, we can introduce new ones. If we've isolated ourselves, we can join in some group activities. And if we're tired, we can give ourselves permission to say no and to have time alone. We might also examine our expectations and remember that special days are not copies of earlier ones. Each is new.

In the holidays ahead, I will continue to do the things that have been special. I will abandon any pattern that gives me no joy.

December 18

The only limit to our realization of tomorrow will be our doubts of today. Let us move forward with strong and active faith.
— *Franklin Delano Roosevelt*

Major changes in our lives may stun us — with delight or perhaps disbelief. After all, not all changes are negative. But when the change is negative, when illness is diagnosed or when pain pervades each day, we may begin to doubt our own inner resources. Once physically strong, we will have to dig deeper than ever to tap into our spiritual resources as well.

If we have doubts today, it may be because we are still locked into our physical selves. We are more than body, and it is our spirits that can be nourished by our caring Higher Power. Our value and importance are revealed by that care. Knowing this, we can move forward with our lives.

I will look beyond my physical body for a source of strength and care.

*Life is not merely living but living in
health.*

— *Martial*

Living in health may seem impossible
for the chronically ill. After all, we reason, it's difficult to live in health if we are
sick.

In fact, living in health is an old-
fashioned term, almost like a benedic-
tion. These days we want to experience the
wellness that goes beyond physical health
by emphasizing emotional and spiritual
health. For the first time we can allow ourselves the right to wellness despite physical illness.

Even with an on-going illness, most of
us don't have constant pain or discomfort.
There are many times we enjoy ourselves.
Playing cards, gardening, going for a
walk, praying, meditating — these activities exercise all of our being — physically,
emotionally, and spiritually.

*I will consider my wellness, not illness, my life
goal.*

December 20

Change does not change tradition. It strengthens it. Change is a challenge and an opportunity, not a threat.
— *Prince Philip*

At holiday times and anniversaries and birthdays, we may lament, "I can't entertain anymore. I just don't have the room. I don't have the strength either." Is what we are telling ourselves really true? Are our friends and families so shallow that they come to our homes only for roast beef or turkey? Do we really have to give up the joy of having company?

Quickly we recognize the nonsense of such thoughts and cope with this situation in the same way we have with so many others — we change and we adapt. We can still welcome our loved ones into our homes. In the simpler meals and the casual atmosphere, our friends and family will find what they have come for — assurance that we still value their company.

I will serve my guests as always — with love and fellowship.

*To know after absence the familiar
street and road and village and house
is to know again the satisfaction of
home.*

— *Hal Borland*

Home is a word that carries all kinds
of meanings for us. For the majority,
home has always been our anchor — the
place where we can go even when we have
had the worst possible of all days. Home
usually means love, but it certainly means
security and comfort.

As the years go by we understand that
home has little to do with a physical structure. It can be a tiny apartment or an elab-
orate mansion. Or — better still — it can
be the special comfort and security we feel
within ourselves. It is, after all, what we
bring to it and to the people around us.
Home is, and always has been, where our
heart is.

*My home acts as one of the roots of my life, and
it has all the qualities that I bring to it.*

December 22

*What's a joy to the one is a nightmare
to the other. That's how it is today,
that's how it will be forever.*
— Bertolt Brecht

Different strokes for different folks is a popular cliche, but it's also an absolute truth when it comes to knowing people. Each of us has our own level of comfort for the activities we do and the performances we give in our lives.

We also find different levels of joy in our spiritual, social, and emotional experiences. Often, we find what we're looking for — what we wish to find — in each situation. What's most important is that we are able to find our own level of joy — wherever we are at that time — and claim it as belonging to us.

My joy may not be the same as someone else's joy, but I shall struggle on to keep the meaning of my joy alive.

*It is a great piece of skill to know how
to guide your luck even while waiting
for it.*

— *Balstar Gracian*

Manipulation sounds like such a harsh
word, but consider the hands of a sur-
geon, the moves of an artist, the skill of an
electrician. They manipulate their physical environment. In doing so, they are
creating. In some subtle way — perhaps
we are not even aware that we are doing it
— we learn to manipulate our lives. We,
too, are very creative.

Some people are able to reach for positive goals, even during seemingly negative
times. These people are capable of scoop-
ing out the very best of life. Those are the
ones who have learned the delicate art of
helping themselves. They can create their
own luck.

*Sometimes luck isn't always caused by a draw
of the cards. I work hard in all areas to improve
my lot, to improve my relationships, to improve
my life.*

December 24

*I have been sick and I have found out,
only then, how lonely I am. Is it too
late?*

— *Eudora Welty*

At one time, we may have thought in
absolute terms. Either a person was our
best friend or not. Things were right or
wrong. We may have driven people from
us — people we could have loved and who
would have enriched our lives.

We have learned that if we are not
happy, we need not accept things as they
stand. The first step is always to admit
there is a problem. Whether it's loneliness, or we have been too brusque with
others, or we need a spiritual change, we
can admit it and do whatever is necessary
to improve. We can turn to friends or
even professionals for help if we need it.
We can do this because it's never too late.

*Although the very thought of change is frighten-
ing, I will assess my life and begin anew today.*

All living souls welcome whatsoever
they are ready to cope with. . . .
                    — *George Santayana*

So often, a problem would be overwhelming if we had to solve it all at once.
We can allow ourselves to dwell only on
small pieces of the problem at one time.
Then, when we've come to terms with one
part, another portion can be dealt with.
Whether we are facing the death of a loved
one or having to cope with other personal
problems, our minds help us sort out the
order in which we can best handle our
pain.

Sometimes, we insist on tackling all of
the problem, and we think ourselves into
a kind of numbness. We're unable to act.
At those times, perhaps we can remind
ourselves of how our minds work best. If
we do, we can let go of the whole situation
and, instead, take on only the small part
we're strong enough to handle.

Today, I will let go of all I'm trying to cope with.
I will pick one or two small, positive things I can
do. Then, I will do them.

December 26

Never let life's hardships disturb you.
After all, no one can avoid problems,
not even saints or sages.
— *Nichiren Daishonen*

A worry-free life. Wouldn't that be the ticket? It's hard to even imagine what life would be like with no problems. Once in a while a person will say, ''If only I'd known . . . I never would have.'' Or, ''If I had understood, I should have. . . .''

We can't live life always regretting past mistakes, and we shouldn't fear future ones either. The key to survival is not maintaining a stiff upper lip, as we have been told, but to express our vulnerability. Stoicism gets nothing but more stress, so we're learning to acknowledge our hardships as they come along. We're not complaining or whining. We're just bonding ourselves to the rest of the human race.

I can face new problems, not because I'm so strong, but because I can honestly admit my weaknesses.

For age is opportunity no less
Than youth itself, though in
another dress,
And as evening twilight fades away
the sky is filled with stars,
invisible day.
　　　— *Henry Wadsworth Longfellow*

As young children we probably had favorite elderly people who made us feel special. We never gave much thought to their age. During young adulthood, however, we may have begun to dread getting older. For some reason we saw the outward signs of aging as the beginning of the end.

As we become wiser and more mature, we come to realize that we once again venerate elderly people — for their wisdom, for their love, for their skills, and especially, for their joy of living. Many of us seem to choose one or two special people whom we wish to be like. And then we try our hardest to measure up.

I look forward to the wisdom and joy of living that often come with age. I am no longer afraid.

December 28

Sadness flies away on the wings of time.

— *Jean De La Fontaine*

When we're sad, it's hard to believe that time will heal all our wounds. An old family-practice doctor used to call it the TOT Treatment — Tincture of Time.

Our sadness may be due to a change in living patterns or even in the weather. It might be due to loss of a loved one, of good health, or even of a cherished object. And our grief takes time.

Whatever the reason for our sadness, after a self-imposed period of time alone, we begin to venture out once again into our world. We work our way, ever so slowly, back into some pattern of normalcy. TOT has done its work once again. Laughter surfaces, and we know we have put enough time and space between us and our sadness. We are whole again.

A time of sadness is natural, just as natural as the rediscovered joy that follows it.

The proper function of man is to live,
not to exist. I shall not waste my days
in trying to prolong them.
— *Jack London*

We are on a remarkable journey that holds wonderful possibilities. Sometimes people who have undergone a crisis think they have arrived at the end of the journey. The excitement of living decreases each day.

Surrounding ourselves with loving, caring people gives us the greatest chance of coming out of the depression caused by our problems. Also, treating ourselves gently can improve our outlook. When we show loving care for others and ourselves, we will once again be moving back into the mainstream of life. We will be filled once again with the excitement and joy of the journey that lies ahead.

I owe myself the excitement of each day to come. Today, I will savor my life.

December 30

To forgive is the highest, most beautiful form of love. In return, you will receive untold peace and happiness.
— *Robert Muller*

When we are trying to cope with a newly diagnosed illness, feelings may be hurt a little too easily, especially when we feel slighted by the very people we feel should understand. We probably are more vulnerable to hurt at first, and we may even at times feel sorry for ourselves.

There comes a time, however, when we can see the futility of carrying old grudges. There's no longer a need to know or prove who was right and who was wrong. As we've learned to cope with our illness, we've become emotionally stronger — strong enough to let go of anger and to forgive. The more we forgive, the calmer and more serene we will become, until ultimately our reward will be inner peace and trust.

I can let go of past hurts. I can bridge the gap caused by misunderstandings.

*Afflictions are not really a good gift —
neither they nor their consequences.
However, if afflictions do come, it is
well that we convert them into afflictions of love. Herein lies the power of
man.*

— *Chaim Nachman Bialik*

All around us we hear cries of "Happy
New Year," and we wonder if this next
year is going to be happier than last year
was. Carrying the burden of chronic pain
or a chronic illness is far more demanding
than most people can imagine. It can
overwhelm our days.

We alone have the power to convert
that pain, loneliness, and any feelings
of guilt into external expressions of ourselves, such as helping others. It's almost
impossible to be completely wound up in
ourselves when we are doing for others.

*I feel positive thoughts about this New Year. My
goal is to reach out to at least one person each
day.*

Peace rises like dawn in the hearts of hope. . . .

Peace reaches from warm and welcoming houses when workers go home.

Peace wraps congregations as worship comes to comforting conclusions. . . .

Peace floats like music through cabin windows to porch-sitters outside.

Peace shimmers from lake water on star-dashed extravagant nights. . . .

Peace blesses the day's end, in the Dylan Thomas way: "I turned the gas down. I got into bed. I said some words into the close and holy darkness, and then I slept."

And so the last page turns to the new page, and we wish the world a happy new year. In peace.

This excerpt is from an editorial written by Ann Daly Goodwin which appeared in the St. Paul Pioneer Press Dispatch *on December 31, 1986.*

INDEX

Other titles that will interest you . . .

Living with a Chronic Illness

by Daniel J. Anderson, Ph.D.

Can we find better ways to cope with chronic illness? Dr. Anderson, President Emeritus of Hazelden, believes we can if we follow the self-care role model established by Alcoholics Anonymous. Chronic illnesses can be faced with better results when the self-help group process becomes an integral part of medical treatment and daily maintenance. 44 pp.
Order No. 5378

Facing a Catastrophic Illness with Hope

by Holly B.

This is the story of a courageous woman who was able to face cancer, chemotherapy and the threat of death with the help of the same Twelve Steps she uses in her chemical dependency recovery program. This woman found the hope that is available to all of us facing a chronic illness. 20 pp.
Order No. 5340
